THE PALEO PRIMER:
A SECOND HELPING

FITTER – HAPPIER – HEALTHIER

Keris Marsden and Matt Whitmore

Mention of specific companies, organizations, or authorities in this book does not imply endorsement by the author or publisher. Information in this book was accurate at the time researched. The authors received no incentives or compensation to promote the item recommendations in the book.
The Paleo Primer: A Second Helping was adapted from the book *Fitter Food: A Second Helping*, written by Keris Marsden and Matt Whitmore, Fitter Food, Inc., and published in the United Kingdom by Ebury Publishing in 2015.

Library of Congress Control Number: 2016937152
Library of Congress Cataloging-in-Publication Data is on file with the publisher
Marsden, Keris 1980- ; and Whitmore, Matt 1985-
The Paleo Primer: A Second Helping/Keris Marsden and Matt Whitmore
ISBN: 9781939563323
1. Cooking 2. Health 3. Diet 4. Low carb

UK Proofreader/Editor: Jane Davis
US Proofreader: Tim Tate
Index: Tim Tate
Book Design: Katherine Keeble (UK)
Production: Caroline De Vita (US)
US Cover Design: Janée Meadows
Illustrations: Mark Goodhead
Photography by Keris Marsden and Matt Whitmore

Published in the United States by Primal Blueprint Publishing
1641 S. Rose Ave., Oxnard, CA 93033

Visit our website at www.primalblueprintpublishing.com. For information on quantity discounts, please call 888-774-6259 or email info@PrimalBlueprintPublishing.com

DISCLAIMER

The ideas, concepts, and opinions expressed in this book are intended to be used for educational purposes only. This book is sold with the understanding that the authors and publisher are not rendering medical advice of any kind, nor is this book intended to replace medical advice, nor to diagnose, prescribe, or treat any disease, condition, illness, or injury. It is imperative that before beginning any diet or exercise program, including any aspect of the diet or exercise methodologies mentioned in *The Paleo Primer: A Second Helping*, you receive full medical clearance from a licensed physician. The authors and publisher claim no responsibility to any person or entity for any liability, loss, or damage caused or alleged to be caused directly or indirectly as a result of the use, application or interpretation of the material in this book. If you object to this disclaimer, you may return the book to publisher for a full refund.

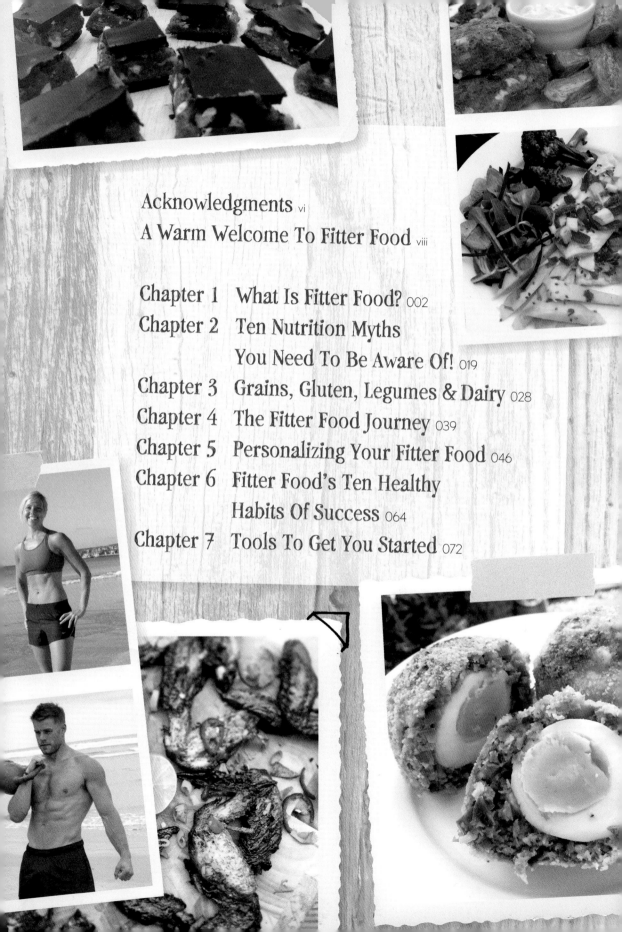

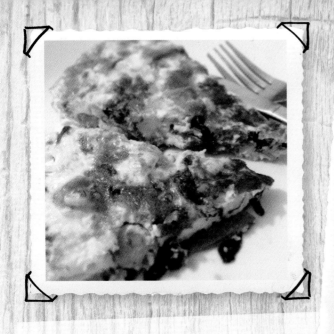

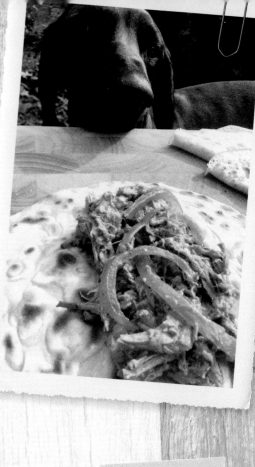

Recipes

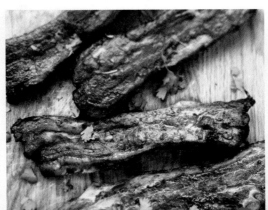

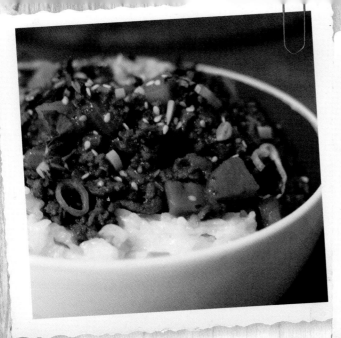
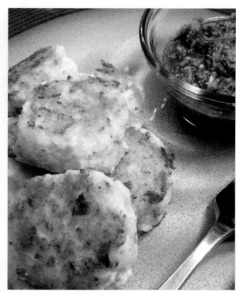

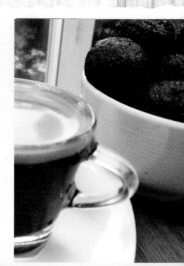

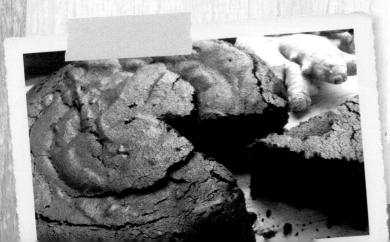

v

ACKNOWLEDGMENTS

We like to place our acknowledgments at the front of the book because *Fitter Food: A Second Helping* wouldn't be here without this awesome bunch. The design, illustrations, recipes and content were a true team effort, not to mention the support we received from our families and the Fitter Food Team. We're so grateful to everyone who contributed.

CLAIRE HARDING
FITTER FOOD TEAM

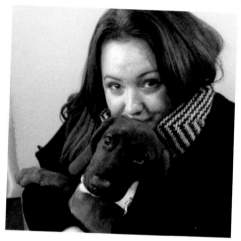

LEGENDARY LYNNE WELCH
FITTER FOOD TEAM

CAROLINE & BOBBY YOUNG
FITTER FOOD TEAM

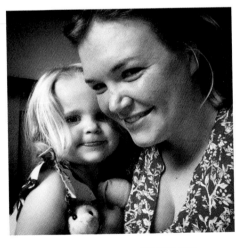

KATHERINE KEEBLE
BOOK DESIGNER

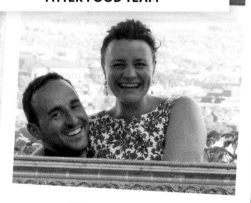

EMMA MIHILL
EXPERT REVIEW

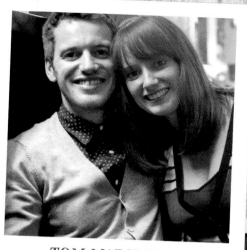

**TOM MARSDEN &
MEGAN CLATWORTHY**
IMAGE DESIGN AND REVIEW

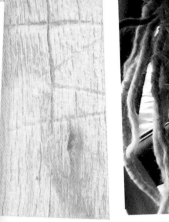

JANE DAVIS
PROOFREADING & EDITING
WWW.COMMCATE.COM

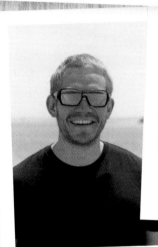

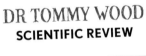

TASHA D'CRUZ
MACRONUTRIENT CALCULATIONS

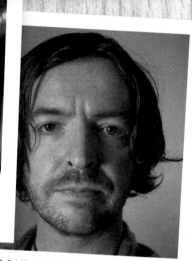

DR TOMMY WOOD
SCIENTIFIC REVIEW

MARK GOODHEAD
ILLUSTRATOR
WWW.MARKGOODHEAD.COM

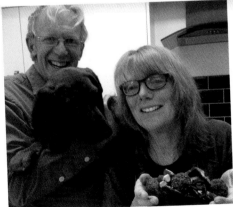

CELINE & CHRIS
KERIS'S AMAZING MOM & DAD

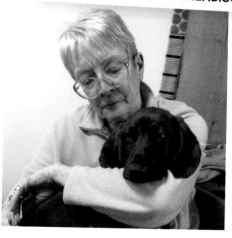

CHRIS
MATT'S LOVELY MOM

www.fitterfood.com

www.twitter.com/fitter_food

www.instagram.com/fitterfood

www.facebook.com/fitterfood

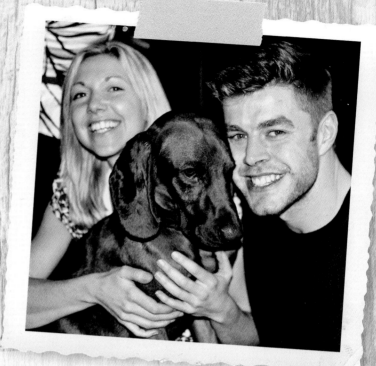

A WARM WELCOME
TO FITTER FOOD

We'd like to take this opportunity to give you a very warm welcome to the Fitter Food community and to say a huge thank you for purchasing our second book. It really means a great deal to us that you have placed your trust in us, and—more importantly—that you have made an investment in yourself.

If you are here because you already have our first book *Fitter Food: A Lifelong Recipe for Health & Fat Loss* (or the US published version, *The Paleo Primer*), we promise more of the same awesome content. If you haven't seen our first book, be sure to check it out; it's packed with practical nutrition and fat loss advice as well as over 100 other delicious recipes to fuel your health journey.

We would also like to assure you that your investment in this book has been a wise one. No matter what your goal(s) are, the principles outlined in this book will support you in achieving and sustaining them. This includes fat loss, elevated energy levels, improved mood, glowing skin, increased performance, better recovery, more confidence and less bloating. The list is endless! If you use the nutrition guidance, adopt the key lifestyle habits we outline, and of course cook the fantastic meals, you WILL look and feel amazing. We suppose you could say the return on your investment will be priceless ☺

We look forward to being a part of your journey and wish you all the success in the world.

THE PALEO PRIMER:
A SECOND HELPING

CHAPTER 1

What Is Fitter Food?

Fitter Food considers itself to be **"Paleo-ish,"** as we believe most people benefit from basing the foundation of their nutrition on the paleo diet. This is simply because it includes some of the most nutritious foods available to us today, focusing on **meat, fish, poultry, eggs, dairy products, vegetables, fruits, nuts, seeds, herbs and spices**.

That said, we're not living in caves, and totally understand that in order to make your nutrition enjoyable and sustainable, you might wish to step out of the caveman zone. The Fitter Food foundation allows you to create a diet that you can complement with a selection of modern-day foods. Many of these can offer some nutritional benefits. And they just might be **a little of what you fancy.** ☺

Being a bit more 'ish' with your paleo also allows you to continually diversify your nutritional intake. This has been shown to benefit the body from a disease-prevention perspective.[1] Furthermore, mankind has always sought new gourmet experiences and adapted consumption in accordance with seasonal variations.

Most importantly, the greater the variety of ingredients in your culinary repertoire, the more creative you can be with your recipe collection, keeping this healthy eating business feeling fresh, exciting and easy to sustain as a way of life.

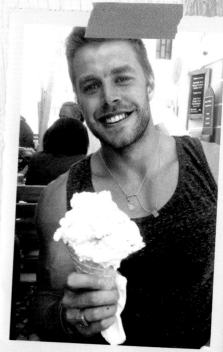

THE CASE FOR FITTER FOOD

THE PROBLEM

With every decade that passes, we continue to migrate further towards an existence where we move and sleep less and less and rely increasingly on industrially processed foods for sustenance. The more technological advances we experience, the more we overwhelm our brains by subjecting them to constant online interaction and information overload. Despite the fact the human body needs sunlight for optimal health to support our vitamin D levels, we barely step out of doors. This causes us to be immune-suppressed and depressed. In short, we're tired, wired and susceptible to illness. This is essentially just surviving, not thriving.

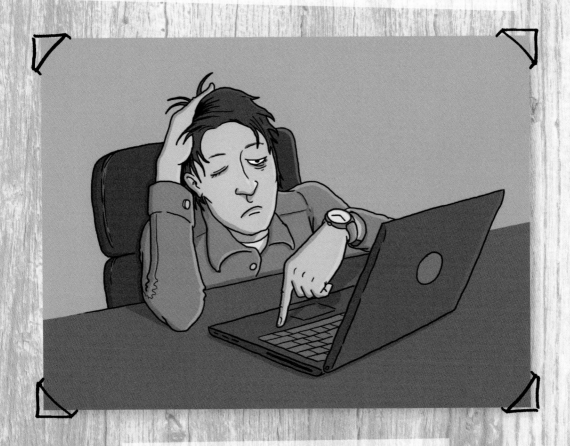

"Let me Google that for you; I only have a million other jobs to do."

THE CONSEQUENCES

A simple way to understand the implications of our modern lifestyle is to consider the human body as being similar to a tree. A tree needs to be nourished from its roots with mineral-rich soil, water and sunlight. If it is starved of any these nutrients it cannot continue to grow, flourish or protect itself from disease. The leaves and branches will begin to rot before the whole tree eventually dies. Your leaves and branches might be suffering already because you have deprived your body of its basic needs. These include:

- ★ Clean water (hydration)
- ★ Sleep
- ★ Nutrient-dense food
- ★ Fresh air
- ★ Chillout time
- ★ Daily movement

Without these, we increase our risk of chronic diseases and symptoms of ill-health:

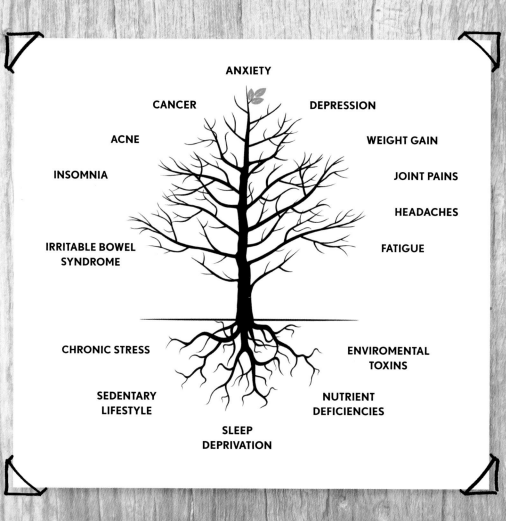

ANXIETY

CANCER

DEPRESSION

ACNE

WEIGHT GAIN

INSOMNIA

JOINT PAINS

HEADACHES

IRRITABLE BOWEL
SYNDROME

FATIGUE

CHRONIC STRESS

ENVIROMENTAL
TOXINS

SEDENTARY
LIFESTYLE

NUTRIENT
DEFICIENCIES

SLEEP
DEPRIVATION

ADDING INSULT TO INJURY

You're stressed and tired, so you turn to modern medicine for help. However, the problem here is that while conventional medicine can work life-saving miracles in an emergency, its approach to resolving more persistent health issues focuses on treating the disease symptoms rather than assessing you as an individual and searching for the root causes of your ill health. It draws upon research-based practice and clinical trials to apply medical solutions. Backed by a powerful pharmaceutical industry, there's pretty much a pill or potion for every problem these days. The issue is that this model of healing is so far from what the founders of conventional medicine intended.

In fact, the man described as the "Father of Western Medicine" was Hippocrates (c.460-c.370 BC). He revolutionized medicine by establishing it as a discipline. Check out some of his awesome quotes here—if he was around today he'd definitely be a Fitter Foodie!

HIPPOCRATES'S TOP 5 TIPS

1 "Walking is man's best medicine."

2 "Natural forces within us are the true healers of disease."

3 "Healing is a matter of time, but it is sometimes also a matter of opportunity."

4 "If we could give every individual the right amount of nourishment and exercise, not too little and not too much, we would have found the safest way to health."

5 "Let food be thy medicine and medicine be thy food."

Despite the origins of modern medicine acknowledging the contribution of healthy exercise, nutrition and lifelong health habits, these are rarely featured in prescriptions today.

Couple this with the fact that every trip to the supermarket involves aisle-upon-aisle of calorie dense, industrially processed foods with added chemicals and ingredients actively designed to encourage addiction to a brand and promote overeating. Possibly even worse are the multiple aisles offering low-fat, light, diet, zero, low-carb, low-calorie or sugar-free foods. In essence, we have ended up with:

A health industry that is not interested in food and a food industry that is not interested in health.

More holistic approaches to health are now developing, which include Functional and Integrative Medicine. These recognize biochemical individuality and the need for more personalized medicine. Instead of the more conventional approach, they view disease as multifactorial, and seek to assess both the internal and external environments of the human body. In doing so, they acknowledge the crucially important roles played by stress, sleep, nutrition, psychological wellbeing and genetics in health and vitality. At some point we hope the medical system will shift towards this more organic approach to health and disease prevention.

YOUR SOLUTION

In the meantime, you can take control of this situation and stop looking for a drug to make you feel better or a food item to help you lose weight. Take advice from one of our all-time favorite films, *Back to the Future*:

"Make like a tree and leave..."

...this all behind! Educate yourself about the fundamentals of human health detailed over the next few chapters, and take control of your body. Fuel it with nutritious food, sensible amounts of sleep, daily exercise and regular stress management.

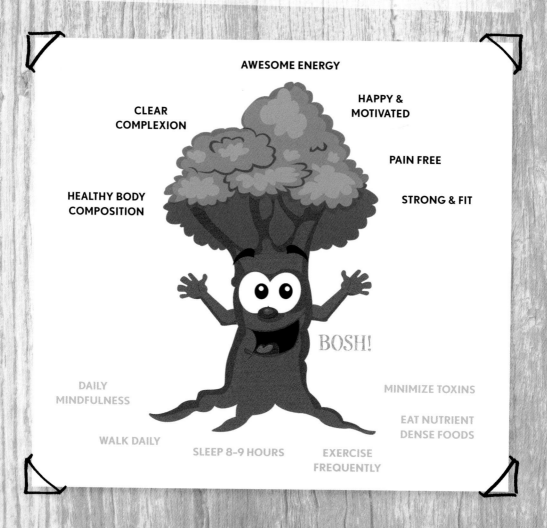

AWESOME ENERGY

HAPPY & MOTIVATED

CLEAR COMPLEXION

PAIN FREE

HEALTHY BODY COMPOSITION

STRONG & FIT

BOSH!

DAILY MINDFULNESS

MINIMIZE TOXINS

EAT NUTRIENT DENSE FOODS

WALK DAILY

SLEEP 8-9 HOURS

EXERCISE FREQUENTLY

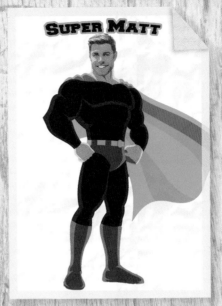

SUPER MATT

Nourishing your own roots with the essential components of health will ensure that the leaves on your tree always look awesome. We're here to help you every step of the way with all the practical information you need, the latest scientific research and lots of knowledge bombs sourced from our own collective experience working with thousands of people in the Fitter Food community.

THE NEED FOR NUTRIENT DENSITY

These recent changes that have taken place in our nutrition, environment and lifestyle have fuelled an increase in cardiovascular disease, cancer, obesity and type 2 diabetes. However, we are not victims here. As the links between diet and chronic disease are becoming clearer, it seems that in our fight to stay **FITTER**:

Nutrition is our most powerful tool. [2]

We encourage you to consider the nutritional density of the food you eat. Everything we consume has the ability to support or hinder our chances of leading a happy, healthy, long life. In order to function optimally, the human body needs vitamins, minerals, antioxidants, protein, fats (including saturated, monounsaturated and polyunsaturated fatty acids) and carbohydrates. Essentially the majority of your nutrition should serve to **bring out the best in you**, as per the sliding scale below:

★ 80-90% of your intake   ★ 10-20% of your intake

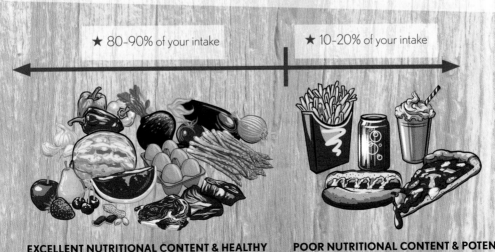

EXCELLENT NUTRITIONAL CONTENT & HEALTHY   **POOR NUTRITIONAL CONTENT & POTENTIALLY HARMFUL IF OVER-CONSUMED**

NUTRIENT DENSITY: THE BOSH INDEX

Many public health guidelines emphasize the concept of healthy food as something that is low in problematic ingredients, for example refined sugar, rather than emphasizing the beneficial nutrients. Numerous attempts have been made to establish a system that can quantify nutrient density outside of government recommendations. These systems use various parameters to assess the macronutrient and micronutrients per calorie or calculate nutrient ratios. The nutrient density approach is our favorite as we believe it's vital to improve nutrition education and empower people with the information they need to support their nutritional needs. However, the scoring systems often have an element of bias towards plant-based foods or have an underlying agenda to sell specific products. With this in mind we used the USDA Nutrient Database to put together our own BOSH Index (BOSH stands for Body Of A Super Human). We assessed the essential amino acids, essential fatty acids, fiber, carbohydrate density and micronutrients per calorie.[3] We also considered the impact on hormone health, antioxidant capacity, prebiotic effect (to support gut health), cost, availability and the pleasure factor. ☺ We suggest you feature these on your Fitter Food table each week due to the abundance of nutrients they contain and the contribution they can make towards optimal health.

FITTER TOP 5

Contain a healthy balance of macronutrients, are high in micronutrients, low in potential toxins and low-cost.

1 Liver
2 Sardines
3 Eggs
4 Sauerkraut
5 Avocados

TOP 5 SOURCES OF FATS
1 Grass-fed butter
2 Avocados
3 Almonds and hazelnuts
4 Cocoa
5 Coconut

TOP 5 SOURCES OF CARBOHYDRATES
1 Sweet potatoes
2 Berries
3 Root vegetables
4 Legumes
5 White potatoes

TOP 5 SOURCES OF MICRONUTRIENTS
1 Herbs: rosemary, basil, thyme and parsley.
2 Spices: cinnamon, turmeric, coriander seed, fennel seeds and chili powder.
3 Bone broth.
4 Dark green leafy vegetables: kale, spinach, arugula and watercress.
5 Cruciferous vegetables and their seeds: broccoli, broccoli sprouts cabbage, Brussels sprouts, mustard greens and mustard seeds.

TOP 5 SOURCES OF PROTEIN
1 Liver
2 Eggs
3 Salmon & sardines
4 Lamb
5 Grass-fed beef

THE BOSH BONUS 10
These foods didn't make our top 5 lists but they still pack a nutrient punch that makes them worthy of a mention.

1 **Seafood:** essential amino acids, B vitamins, zinc, iodine and selenium.
2 **Garlic:** prebiotic, vitamin B6, manganese, and its sulphur compounds are cardio protective.
3 **Kiwi:** low in sugar, high in fiber, potassium, vitamin C, and transforms a green smoothie.
4 **Bananas:** prebiotic, potassium, cheap, convenient and tasty.
5 **Coffee:** antioxidant polyphenols, prebiotic and it's COFFEE!

6 **Sea vegetables:** iodine, magnesium, manganese and iron.
7 **Green tea:** prebiotic, antioxidant polyphenols and L-theanine (which has calming, mood enhancing properties).
8 **High-fat dairy:** essential amino acids, probiotic bacteria, conjugated linoleic acid, omega-3 fatty acids and fat-soluble vitamins A, E, K and K2.
9 **Tomatoes:** vitamin C, potassium, vitamin K, and rich in the antioxidant lycopene.
10 **Pork:** essential amino acids, B vitamins, iron, zinc, selenium, and it's where bacon comes from. ☺

THE PALEO PRIMER PYRAMID

To help you fully understand the principles we advocate, we've built a Paleo Primer pyramid as an illustration of how you can structure your food intake. It demonstrates how you can prioritize consumption of a nutrient-dense foundation and then build in some options based upon your personal preference, current health status, training routine, lifestyle and of course your goals.

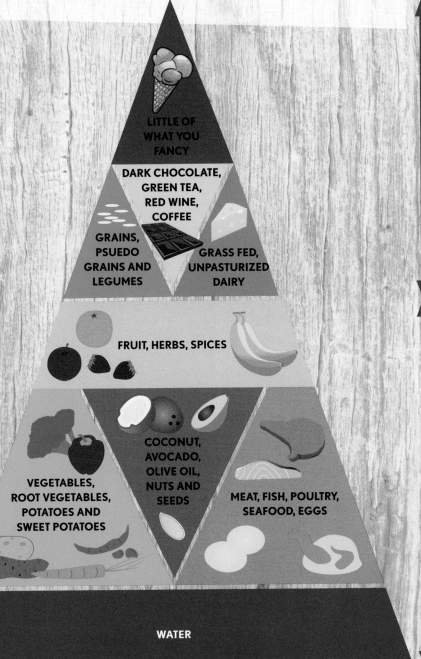

OPTIONAL

FOUNDATION

LITTLE OF WHAT YOU FANCY

DARK CHOCOLATE, GREEN TEA, RED WINE, COFFEE

GRAINS, PSUEDO GRAINS AND LEGUMES

GRASS FED, UNPASTURIZED DAIRY

FRUIT, HERBS, SPICES

VEGETABLES, ROOT VEGETABLES, POTATOES AND SWEET POTATOES

COCONUT, AVOCADO, OLIVE OIL, NUTS AND SEEDS

MEAT, FISH, POULTRY, SEAFOOD, EGGS

WATER

THE FIVE ESSENTIAL INGREDIENTS THAT MAKE IT FITTER

The following attributes are what really make Paleo Primer work its magic once it's inside your body:

1. Fitter Food Is Gut Friendly Food

The importance of gut health cannot be underestimated. No matter what your health goal, whether it is fat loss, hormonal balance, immune support or increased energy and enhanced performance, each of these starts within the digestive system. Firstly, the digestive tract is where you begin to break down all the awesome Fitter Food you've eaten. Secondly, the bacteria located in the colon are involved in a number of essential functions, including:

★ Vitamin production
★ The regulation of hormones and neurotransmitters (brain chemicals)
★ Detoxification
★ Immune defense

In fact, our entire body acts as a host to trillions of bacteria. They sit on our skin, inside our mouth, ears, nose, airways and a large proportion reside in the digestive tract. For every human gene in your body, there are 100 more bacterial genes as they outnumber our own cells by 10 to 1. In other words you could say we're 90% bacteria and only 10% human.[4] This is referred to as your 'microbiome' and plays a fundamental role in your overall health.

Keeping these little guys safe and nourished is really the key to being a happy and healthy human being. If we don't support this army of beneficial bacteria, then less desirable bacteria, pathogenic yeasts and viruses will seize the opportunity to invade. These will trigger a cascade of inflammation as our immune system becomes chronically activated, depleting nutrients, energy and wellness.

Our gut bacteria thrive on food in its natural state with minimal processing, so all of the natural fats, connective tissue and fiber have been retained. If you don't recognize an ingredient, then the chances are that your gut bacteria won't either. It seems they're also not fans of many man-made foodstuffs such as additives, preservatives, emulsifiers, sweeteners and even flours.[5]

In our first book we detail the benefits of following an elimination diet if you have a damaged digestive system, and focusing on a paleo foundation to support digestive repair and the return of healthy gut function.

As well as eliminating processed foods, it's also vital to feed your little army of bacteria to help it thrive. Certain nutrients help gut bacteria to proliferate and encourage the growth of different beneficial strains of bacteria. The more diverse the balance of your bacteria is, the more protection it offers you against certain diseases.[6]

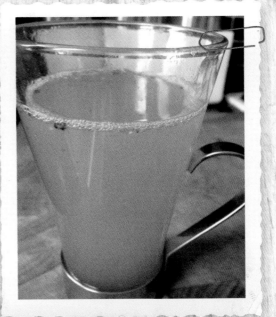

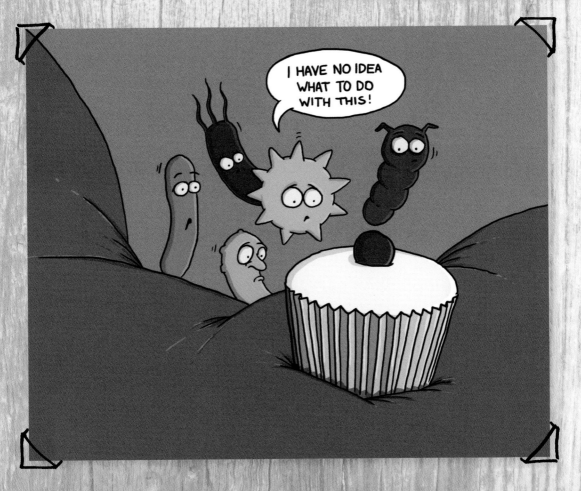

The following are what we consider gut superfoods due to their ability to support digestive function. You should aim to include them on a regular basis on your Fitter Food menu.

GUT SUPERFOOD	EXAMPLES	FUNCTION
★ Unpasteurized, fermented foods	Kimchi, sauerkraut, kombucha, kefir	These are lacto-fermented; a process that allows probiotic bacteria to naturally culture on the food. If consumed regularly they support a healthy balance of gut bacteria.[7]
★ Bone broth (see page 209)	Chicken, beef or lamb	Cooking bones for prolonged periods creates a broth rich in proteins that nourish the gut, including glycine, which stimulates the production of stomach acid[8] and glutamine, which supports the integrity of the gastrointestinal tract.[9]
★ Organ meats	Liver, heart, tongue, sweetbreads	Packed with the essential micronutrients that support healthy digestive function including vitamin A, zinc and iron.[10]
★ Prebiotic foods	Onions, leeks, garlic, artichokes, asparagus, root vegetables, cabbage	Prebiotic foods skip absorption in the small intestine and upon reaching the colon provide nutrition for our gut bacteria. Regular consumption promotes the proliferation and activity of beneficial bacteria.[11]
★ Short and medium chain fatty acids	Butter, ghee and coconut oil	These fats fuel and protect the cells and bacteria in our gut so they can exert an anti-inflammatory effect and regulate healthy gut function.[12] The lauric acid in coconuts has an antimicrobial and anti-fungal effect.[13]
★ Sour foods	Apple cider vinegar, lemon juice, unpasteurized pickles	These have been used across traditional cultures as digestive aids supporting the role of stomach acid and digestive enzymes.[14] These sour foods are also acidic and have the potential to slow down the digestion of carbohydrates, reducing the release of glucose into the blood stream and the subsequent surge in insulin.[15]
★ Polyphenols	Grapes, green and black tea, coffee, cocoa, berries	The bioactive compounds in polyphenol-rich foods are metabolised by our gut bacteria and support a more beneficial balance.[16]

BASICALLY OUR GUT BACTERIA LOVE CHOCOLATE AND COFFEE. ☺

GUT HEALTH & FAT LOSS

Research is increasingly suggesting that the bacteria in our gut may be crucial in addressing the current obesity crisis. Studies comparing the balance of bacteria in obese versus lean individuals have showed significant differences. Slimmer individuals have much more varied strains of bacteria and a wider variety of microbes called bacteroides. These are essential in the process of breaking down plant starch and fiber into short chain fatty acids so they can be used as a source of energy by the body.[17] It seems that gut bacteria may be influencing how we metabolize carbohydrates and burn or store fat. They also affect the production of hunger and satiety hormones.[18]

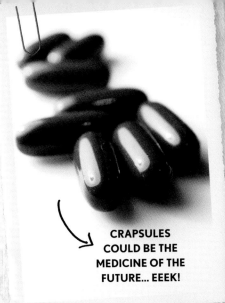

CRAPSULES COULD BE THE MEDICINE OF THE FUTURE... EEEK!

Huge research projects are underway[19] to establish whether we can 'cultivate' fat loss by transferring the bacteria from healthy individuals to obese and overweight via fecal microbiota transplants in order to improve their metabolic health.[20] The results are promising, although we might just stick to sauerkraut and kefir for now.

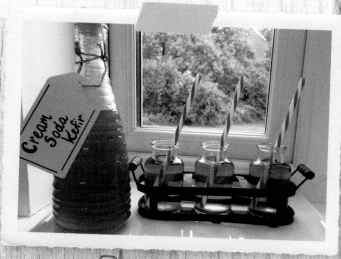

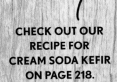

CHECK OUT OUR RECIPE FOR CREAM SODA KEFIR ON PAGE 218.

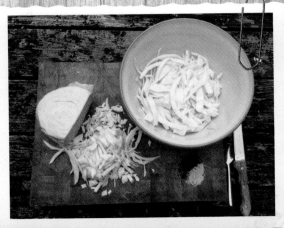

SPEEDY SAUERKRAUT WITH A TWIST PAGE 219.

2. Detoxifying Nutrients

One of the issues causing multiple health problems today is that our detoxification systems are becoming overwhelmed with increasing amounts of pollution, agricultural chemicals in our food, medications and the contamination of our tap water. Many household cleaning products and personal care products are also loaded with compounds that your body may have to work hard to detoxify and get rid of.[21] The Environmental Working Group recently launched the **Skin Deep®** **Cosmetics Database** that allows you to check the ingredients in your own products.[22] Luckily our bodies are well equipped to dispose of toxins they come into contact with, including endotoxins produced internally by bacteria and as a by-product of biological reactions and exotoxins that we are exposed to externally in our food, water and environment.

Nutritional choices play a fundamental role in detoxification because they can either support and enhance our natural detox pathways or simply add to the burden.

The liver is one of the main organs responsible for detoxification. It adopts a two-phase approach to removing toxins from the body. Phase one collects the toxins, including excess hormones, alcohol, caffeine and medications, and prepares them to be removed by putting them through a series of chemical reactions. The second phase of detoxification involves something called 'conjugation,' where the waste products are wrapped up and passed out of the body via the kidneys (through urination) or the digestive system (through bowel movements). If the toxins are not eliminated on a daily basis, they may be reabsorbed back into the body, increasing the toxic load.

A large toxic burden may also cause health issues, so it's important to consume nutrients which support each phase of detoxification: these include protein, antioxidants, vitamins and minerals.

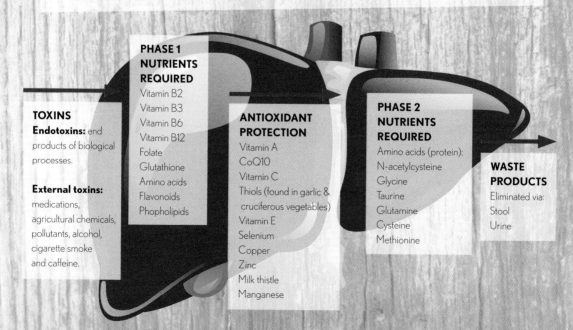

TOXINS
Endotoxins: end products of biological processes.

External toxins: medications, agricultural chemicals, pollutants, alcohol, cigarette smoke and caffeine.

PHASE 1 NUTRIENTS REQUIRED
Vitamin B2
Vitamin B3
Vitamin B6
Vitamin B12
Folate
Glutathione
Amino acids
Flavonoids
Phopholipids

ANTIOXIDANT PROTECTION
Vitamin A
CoQ10
Vitamin C
Thiols (found in garlic & cruciferous vegetables)
Vitamin E
Selenium
Copper
Zinc
Milk thistle
Manganese

PHASE 2 NUTRIENTS REQUIRED
Amino acids (protein):
N-acetylcysteine
Glycine
Taurine
Glutamine
Cysteine
Methionine

WASTE PRODUCTS
Eliminated via:
Stool
Urine

The following foods in particular are rich in the nutrients that actively support each of the phases:

★ Proteins, especially glycine, which is found in organ meats, bone broth and fish skin
★ Cruciferous vegetables: broccoli, cauliflower, Brussels sprouts, mustard seeds
★ Dark green leafy vegetables: kale, spinach, arugula, and watercress
★ Garlic, leeks, onions and apples
★ Egg yolks
★ Green tea
★ Herbs and spices

As you can see, our recipes include many of the above ingredients, making it easy to get a dose of detoxing with a **Pimped** Salad, pages 197-203, Dairy-Free Liver Paté, page 210 or any of the soups from pages 108-117 which are brimming with vegetables, garlic, leeks and onions.

3. Hormone-Friendly Nutrients

A significant part of optimal health is achieving effective communication across the whole body. Our hormones play a significant role in this process and we often liken them to the email system of the body, relaying messages about what tasks need to be done and what the current state of affairs is. It's vital that our body listens and responds to these messages. Imagine if you ignored your inbox for a week; it would be chaos! Insulin is the master hormone, as it plays an essential role in the transportation of nutrients into the cells in the body.

Once the nutrients are inside the cells they can fuel various metabolic processes. However, there is a risk that this step may not take place because our cells may ignore the insulin. In this case, the nutrients you eat may be stored as excess body fat instead, which leaves you gaining weight while your cells are starving. This is known as insulin resistance.

It's important that your nutrition, training and lifestyle support good insulin health and keep your cells responsive to the instructions offered by this hormone. This is known as insulin sensitivity.

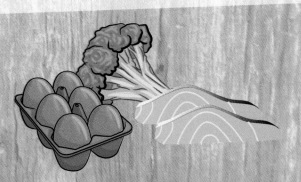

HORMONE-FRIENDLY FOODS

OMEGA-3 RICH FISH

Omega-3 fats sit in the outer membrane of our cells and maintain its fluidity. This enables nutrients to be moved in and out of the cell. For the best sources of omega-3s, think SMASH:

★ Salmon
★ Mackerel
★ Anchovies
★ Sardines
★ Herrings

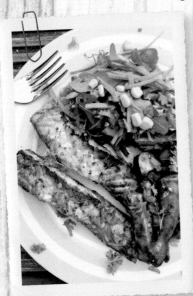

MIGHTY MINERALS

Minerals are hugely important for optimal hormone health. The following minerals are worthy of a special mention. If your nutrition has been lacking for a few years you may also benefit from taking these in supplemental form to catch up. But start with finding them in these yummy foods:

Magnesium-rich foods: dark chocolate, nuts, pumpkin, sesame seeds, spinach, kale, chard, avocados, bananas, bone broth.

Zinc-rich foods: lamb, beef, turkey, shrimp, oysters, cashew nuts, sesame seeds, pumpkin seeds.

Chromium-rich foods: broccoli, sweet potatoes, garlic, eggs, beef, cinnamon.

ANCESTRAL CARBOHYDRATES

Consuming carbohydrates from nature that have not been subjected to processing (i.e. transformed into a liquid or flour) will have less of an impact on blood glucose levels. Good sources include: root vegetables, sweet potatoes, low sugar fruit (berries, avocados, lemons, limes and grapefruit) and non-starchy vegetables.

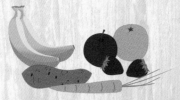

INDULGE IN ANTIOXIDANTS

The following are all rich sources of antioxidants, which help to mop up free radicals that can damage our DNA and decrease insulin sensitivity.

✔ Dark green leafy vegetables like spinach, arugula, kale and watercress
✔ Herbs and spices
✔ Tea, coffee and red wine
✔ Cocoa

Moderation is the key!

4. Quick, Easy, TASTY and Sustainable Nutrition

The problem with healthy eating these days is that most people are either **"on the diet"** or **"off the diet;"** they aren't aiming to find a sustainable model of nutrition and exercise that can be implemented on a long-term basis.

A much more effective and sensible approach to your nutrition should bring the desired health benefits, improve your quality of life and be enjoyable. This will mean that you can continue with it beyond Monday, or whichever day you commence **"The Diet!"** The reality is it shouldn't feel like a diet because this implies a temporary measure. But why would you pursue superior health on a temporary basis? Many of the simple changes we suggest are incredibly easy to implement as daily habits. These include eating a protein-based breakfast instead of sugary cereal, eating zucchini or sweet potatoes in place of refined carbohydrates and cooking your own meals so you can ditch the processed foods that offer no nutritional substance.

If you think health and fat loss is based on shakes or starving yourself, you will never sustain these things. And more than likely, you'll end up faceplanting into a pizza after a couple of weeks of trying to restrain yourself. At Fitter Food, we work hard to develop recipes that are tasty, hearty and hit the spot so that you never feel like you're missing out. We use minimal ingredients and quick cooking methods so you can easily fuel yourself on nutritious, healthy, homemade food; day in, day out.

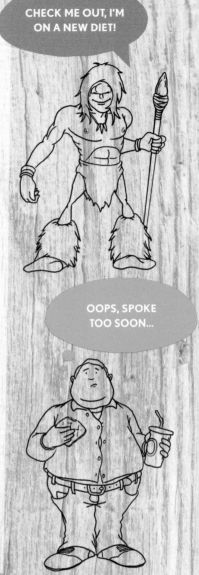

CHECK ME OUT, I'M ON A NEW DIET!

OOPS, SPOKE TOO SOON...

5. Anti-Inflammatory and Immune-Supporting Nutrients

If we fall ill, many of us reach for medications to make ourselves feel better. These tend to work by suppressing the symptoms rather than actually helping your immune system fight the bacterial or viral infection that is making you sick. While these may offer short-term symptom relief, many have undesirable side effects.

Your nutrition and lifestyle can play a huge role in building up your own immune system to protect you against future infections. Poor nutrition, sleep deprivation and chronic stress will all make you susceptible to illness. The following all feature frequently in our Fitter Food recipes and help to build up your natural immune defenses:

"Let Food Be Thy Medicine" — HIPPOCRATES

FERMENTED FOODS

As you now know these are gut superfoods. As it's estimated that 80% of your immune system is located in the digestive tract, building a healthy balance of bacteria helps protect you against any bugs and germs that enter the body.

WHITE OR SWEET POTATOES

Both are a great choice of carbohydrate offering lots of fiber and micronutrients including immune-boosting vitamin C. Sweet potatoes and other orange vegetables also contain beta-carotene, a precursor nutrient for vitamin A which is integral for the health of the skin and the gut, both the first lines of defense for our immune system.[23]

You might be a little puzzled by the suggestion that **white potatoes are good for you!** However, recent reviews have shown that they can be a great addition to a healthy diet[24], as they add variety, improve satiety and are a low cost, traditional ingredient used in a wide variety of dishes. So including them in your nutrition makes life much easier and cheaper! The process of cooking white potatoes and then allowing them to cool increases a type of fiber, known as 'resistant starch,' which literally resists digestion and helps to feed the bacteria in our gut, supporting our immune defense system.[25] Lentils are another good source of resistant starch.

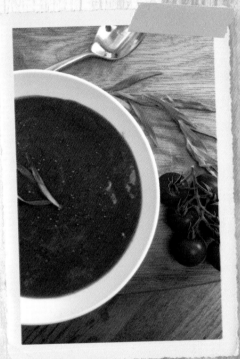

GINGER

Ginger has been used for centuries in Chinese and alternative medicine for its anti-inflammatory effect. An easy way to consume it is to sip on fresh ginger tea throughout the day, or add ginger to soups, smoothies and stir fries. **Broccoli, berries, omega-3 rich fish, green tea and turmeric** also have a similar effect by suppressing the release of inflammatory chemicals.[26]

GARLIC

Garlic enhances immune function by stimulating different types of immune cells including macrophages, lymphocytes and natural killer cells.[27] An important tip with garlic is to chop it up just before cooking and leave it for ten minutes. This allows the enzymes in the garlic to get to work and release the active compound known as allicin. Whenever you're making soup, stews or burgers, chop the garlic first and set aside to let it work its magic.

SOUPS

Soups have the potential to pack an amazing nutrient punch as you can include lots of vegetables, antioxidant rich herbs and spices, garlic and onions. Check out our awesome range on pages 108-117). Making soups with bone broth (see page 209) enhances their immune-boosting and healing properties by adding minerals and collagen to support the immune system.[28]

CHAPTER 2

Ten Nutrition Myths
You Need To Be AWARE Of!

Some recommendations we make in this book might confuse you a little or contradict nutrition advice you have been given in the past. Throughout the 20th century we've been encouraged to count calories and limit saturated fat, cholesterol and salt. We've been actively encouraged by the government to eat more packaged "health foods" created by the food industry, including low-fat spreads, cookies and cereals or calorie-controlled packaged meals that are low in salt. At the same time, chronic diseases have risen exponentially.

Evidence is gradually stacking up that challenges many existing public health recommendations. Extensive reviews of the scientific literature, large scale studies and advances in research technology have helped to establish that many claims surrounding nutrition and disease are completely incorrect and originated from misinterpretations of the data or unsupported hypotheses.

Sadly, despite the overwhelming evidence against these existing guidelines, public health establishments are taking time to revise their recommendations and communicate the updated research. This may be due to a reluctance to take on the powerful food industry, especially given the fact that the majority of the research suggests we should be stepping away from industrially processed convenience foods and moving back to home-cooked meals based on natural ingredients. The following nutrition myths detail some of the false health recommendations that will hopefully be revised in the not-too-distant future.

All government dietary guidance should come with a tobacco-style caution:

"Following this advice could seriously damage your health."

JOANNA BLYTHMAN [29]

MYTH #1
Saturated fat intake is associated with heart disease.

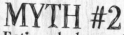

This hypothesis was developed back in the 1940s and once placed under the scrutiny of a large scale, meta-analysis study has finally been disproven. A study published in the *American Journal of Clinical Nutrition* confirmed that **there is no significant evidence to conclude dietary saturated fat is associated with an increased risk of coronary heart disease or cardiovascular disease risk.**[30] Another study recently shared by the UK National Health Service, carried out by leading researchers from renowned academic institutes and funded by the Medical Research Council and British Heart Foundation, concluded that evidence does not support current nutritional guidelines which encourage high consumption of polyunsaturated fatty acids and low consumption of saturated fats, fatty acids and low consumption of saturated fats.[31]

MYTH #2
Eating cholesterol increases your risk of heart disease.

All the latest scientific research strongly suggests that, according to the science, **there is no direct correlation between dietary cholesterol intake and disease risk.**[32] Despite the fact that many countries, including the US, have now updated their dietary guidelines to reflect this research, the general public retains a fear of dietary cholesterol. Only 25% of our blood cholesterol comes from our food; the remaining **75% of cholesterol is produced internally by the liver**. Furthermore, our body regulates blood cholesterol levels closely so if you reduce your intake of cholesterol-rich foods it will simply produce more to make up the difference.[33] You can read more on this topic in Chris Kresser's "Paleo Cure" or "High Cholesterol Action Plan".[34]

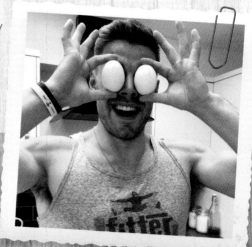

MYTH #3
Red meat consumption increases your risk of inflammatory disease including cardiovascular disease, type 2 diabetes and cancer.

There is insufficient data to suggest that red meat intake is associated with cancer.[35] If anything, conjugated linoleic acid (CLA), which is a natural fat found in beef, has been shown to have cancer protective properties.[36] Greater amounts of CLA are found in grass-fed meats and dairy products.[37] Eating meat has been a fundamental component of human nutrition for thousands of years, yet heart disease, cancer and diabetes have increased significantly in the last 50 years. One theory is that some of the by-products created when we cook meat, known as heterocyclic amines (HCAs) or polycyclic aromatic hydrocarbons (PAHs), could be linked with some inflammatory conditions.[38,39] Cooking methods that expose meat to smoke or charring contribute to the formation of HCAs and PAHs, so well-cooked, grilled or barbecued chicken and steak have higher concentrations of these compounds.[40] However, you can lower the amount in your food by cooking at a lower temperature, making sure you don't burn the meat and marinating the meat in herbs and olive oil before cooking. The antioxidant content of these foods will help protect against carcinogenic compounds.

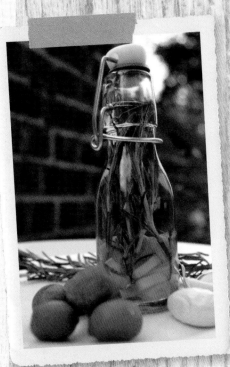

MYTH #4
A high-protein diet puts a strain on the kidneys and raises your risk of kidney disease.

There is no evidence to support any association between a high-protein diet and kidney disease. There is some research to suggest limiting protein intake may be beneficial to individuals with chronic kidney disease. Controlled scientific trials have shown that high-protein diets elicit changes in kidney function.[41] However, further investigation has established that these changes are actually a healthy adaptive response to the additional protein intake.[42] A review of all the published research on high-protein diets and kidney disease concluded that a healthy diet rich in protein does not lead to kidney disease.[43]

MYTH #5
Eating carbohydrates will lead to weight gain, especially if consumed after 6 pm.

If you look at ancestral diets and modern hunter-gatherer tribes, their macronutrient intakes vary widely. Some exist on a higher intake of carbohydrates, while others exist on diets that contain high amounts of saturated fats. One of the most widely-studied modern hunter-gatherer tribes is the Kitavan tribe, based on an island off Papua New Guinea. The Kitavan consume 70% of their calories from carbohydrates, yet are one of the healthiest populations that exist today and do not suffer the same issues of obesity, diabetes and heart disease experienced by industrial societies.[44]

It's imperative you understand:

CARBOHYDRATES DO NOT MAKE YOU FAT!
Now read that again out loud!

However, some unhealthy lifestyle habits like not exercising enough, not sleeping for eight hours a night, chronic stress and eating refined and processed foods can compromise our ability to utilize carbohydrates for energy—so in simple terms they become stored as fat. A recent study suggests that one of the best approaches we can apply to our carbohydrate intake is to preferentially source **most of our carbohydrates from ancestral foods** like root vegetables, sweet potatoes, vegetables and fruit, rather than from anything that comes in a package. These carbohydrates are structured much more naturally with higher amounts of fiber and feed protective bacteria in our gut.[45] In terms of deciding when it is best to eat your carbohydrates, this is influenced by numerous factors including your exercise routine and individual hormone health. Some studies have observed benefits from consuming carbohydrates at breakfast.[46] However, a recent study suggested there may be a health advantage to the majority of your carbohydrate consumption being with evening meals, especially for overweight individuals with a higher risk of developing diabetes or cardiovascular disease. Eating carbohydrates in the evening can help improve daytime hormonal balance, encouraging weight loss and healthy appetite levels throughout the day.[47] Carbohydrates consumed in the evening also support our natural circadian rhythm (sleep and wake cycle) by encouraging the release of our sleep hormone, melatonin, and the calming neurotransmitter serotonin.[48] If you struggle with insomnia or any sleep related disorders, try increasing your intake of carbohydrates at night to see if you can benefit from their sleep-inducing properties.

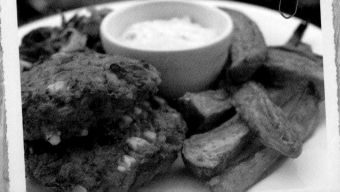

MYTH #6
Vegetable oils and low-fat spreads are good for heart health.

6

The British Heart Foundation and dieticians often recommend soy, sunflower, corn and canola oils as 'heart healthy' options. These vegetable oils gained popularity in the 1960s following claims that saturated fats were responsible for the development of heart disease. Although the hypothesis was never proven **(and has now been disproven—see myth #1)**, many governments and public health institutes began to recommend vegetable oil as the healthiest cooking oil. The use of traditional, minimally processed fats such as lard and butter declined rapidly. The issue here is that vegetable oils are incredibly high in omega-6 fatty acids. Consuming these frequently may disrupt your body's ratio of omega-3 and omega-6 fatty acids and increase your risk of inflammatory diseases, including cardiovascular disease, obesity, cancer and type 2 diabetes.[49][50][51] Meanwhile, the case for putting butter back on the menu just keeps growing! It is a rich source of fat-soluble vitamins including K2[52][53] as well as CLA, which has anti-cancer properties.[54] Not to mention the fact that it's blooming delicious!

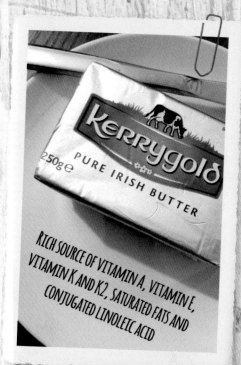

RICH SOURCE OF VITAMIN A, VITAMIN E, VITAMIN K AND K2, SATURATED FATS AND CONJUGATED LINOLEIC ACID

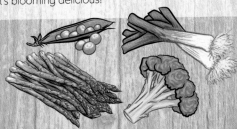

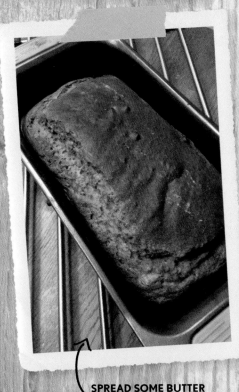

TIP
Add some butter to your green veggies to improve absorption of fat soluble vitamins.

SPREAD SOME BUTTER ON YOUR CHOCOLATE PROTEIN LOAF PAGE 222

MYTH #7
Salt intake needs to be restricted to lower blood pressure and decrease your risk of a heart attack or stroke.

Salt has been vilified over the last few decades as a potential cause of high blood pressure issues. However, scientific research does not actually support this association. The human body also has a basic physiological need for salt, or more specifically for sodium. It plays a significant role in the regulation of fluid balance, nervous system health and cardiovascular function. One exception to this may be individuals with impaired kidney function and salt sensitivity. However, this can easily be balanced with potassium-rich foods (such as bananas, avocados, tomatoes and coconut water) and magnesium-rich foods (like dark chocolate, nuts and green leafy vegetables).

Chris Kresser performed a review of the current salt recommendations and concluded that the scientific data supports a daily intake ranging from 3000 to 7000 milligrams of sodium, or between 1.5 to 3.5 teaspoons of salt, per day. This may vary across age, gender, physical activity levels and health conditions.[55]

Salt can be sourced naturally from foods like celery and seafood, or you can add natural salts like Celtic Sea salt or Himalayan Pink salt to your food. These also provide natural trace minerals. However, it's best to avoid table salt as this undergoes processing and refinement which removes several beneficial nutrients.

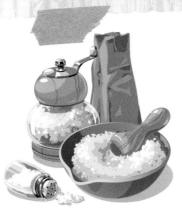

MYTH #8
Eating fat makes you fat

Let's start by making it clear:

FATS DO NOT MAKE YOU FAT! Now read that again out loud!

A comprehensive review recently concluded that fat consumption does not directly increase body fat.[56] Fat will not intrinsically make you fat any more than protein or carbohydrates do. When considering macronutrients, it's important to understand where the confusion arises based on the basic calorie content of macronutrients:

★ Fat = 9 calories per gram
★ Protein = 4 calories per gram
★ Carbohydrates = 4 calories per gram
★ Alcohol = 7 calories per gram

As fat contains the most calories per gram it may be a little easier to consume more calories from fat-based foods, and a low-fat diet will naturally be a little lower in calories. However, because fats exert a satiating effect, they can be hugely effective in supporting weight loss by helping to regulate appetite. One study observed that the consumption of saturated fats, including butter and coconut oil, increased appetite-suppressing hormones and slowed the emptying of the stomach, keeping individuals feeling fuller for longer.[57] It seems that, if left to their natural devices, our bodies are good at compensating for the extra calories we take on board when eating fats. The caveat here is that the fats consumed are from natural sources and not processed junk foods that have the ability to override our satiety signals and actually encourage us to consume more calories than we need.

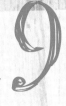

MYTH #9
All calories are created equal: the total amount is what counts and the source is irrelevant.

The food and diet industries have spent years developing calorie-controlled shakes, bars and meals that encourage people to rely on calorie counting as the most effective method of weight management. However, these low-calorie products are also extremely low in nutrients, and not something that our bodies are naturally designed to live on. In fact, if you base your health on simply counting calories and ignore the source, you will likely end up consuming more industrially processed foods because:

a) If we're counting calories, it's much easier to rely on pre-packaged foods that tell us the calorie content. No math required!

b) These products are designed to appeal to our gluttonous instincts with lots of non-food ingredients that add bulk, texture and taste, but leave us always wanting more.

However, there are many potential consequences to relying on reducing calories and eating calorie-controlled foods to improve your body composition. It may have a negative physiological impact upon your body by causing nutrient deficiencies, hormonal imbalances and undesirable changes to the gut microbiome.[58] If this is your only approach to fat loss it could mean you struggle to achieve or sustain any results and end up constantly looking for the next magic solution. It's a great result as far as the diet industry is concerned, as it creates customers for life.

Another argument against the 'calorie is a calorie' claim is the satiety index of foods. One study compared the effectiveness of natural versus processed foods in terms of how they score on a satiety index. Many of the highest-scoring foods that keep you feeling full and satisfied were from natural sources, while the lowest-scoring foods tended to be processed. Boiled potatoes had a seven-fold higher satiety score than a croissant. The satiety score of the food also significantly influenced the amount of food consumed up to two hours after. So the more satisfying the food you eat, the less likely you are to want to snack later![59,60]

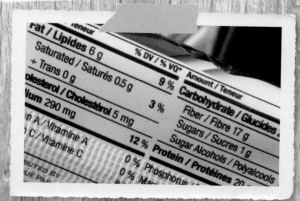

MYTH #10

Losing weight is achieved by eating less and exercising more.

Studies are currently exploring how we've created our current obesity-promoting environment. Essentially, it seems that the modern day environment upsets the natural hormonal communication within the body that is designed to regulate fat mass and keep our body composition healthy.[61] Did you know that your body doesn't want to be overweight? In fact, our bodies are always fighting to survive and thrive, which includes being free from disease and having an optimal amount of body fat.

The human body has mechanisms in place designed to keep us at a healthy weight. We have something known as a **body fat setpoint**. This is the amount of body fat your body has decided is healthy for you and is tightly regulated by hormones. Your body fat is constantly relaying signals to your brain, almost like **'fat feedback,'** to let it know there are adequate fat stores for survival. It does this by producing the hormone leptin.

HYPOTHALAMUS

FOOD INTAKE

ENERGY EXPENDED

LEPTIN

FAT TISSUE

The hormones leptin and insulin are both major players ensuring that the system operates effectively and that fat mass is regulated rather like how a thermostat controls the central heating in a household. If you are underweight, leptin levels will drop. Your brain will detect this and send out instructions to increase calorie absorption in the gut, increase appetite hormones and slow down the rate you burn calories at rest. This will help you to increase fat mass. If leptin levels rise, your brain detects an abundance of body fat and will decrease calorie absorption, lower hunger hormones and increase the rate you utilize calories to help you burn off the excess body fat. You could say we have our own internal **FAT-O-STAT**.

Your body is constantly defending the amount of body fat it thinks is healthy for you based on this fat feedback and the messages it receives from our environment. The problem is that our increasingly sedentary lifestyles and consumption of highly palatable foods confuse the Fat-O-STAT, so it defends a body fat setpoint that is actually too high. Our brains can also sometimes end up ignoring the fat feedback. This scenario is known as **leptin resistance**.

ALWAYS HUNGRY, NEVER FULL?

Processed foods in particular have a dangerous ability to ruin the effectiveness of your Fat-O-STAT by offering an overwhelming sense of food reward that overrides your natural appetite and sense of satiety. The food industry has spent years researching the ingredients that have the ability to activate the reward centers in the brain. It turns out that the combination of salt, fat and sugar is one we just can't resist—and as a result, these are the primary components of most baked goods and junk food.[62]

Don't believe us? Try removing all sense of food reward for a week by eating nothing but boiled potatoes, and watch the weight drop off![63]

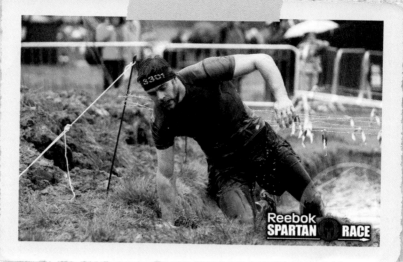

WHAT ABOUT EXERCISE?

As personal trainers we're huge fans of exercise, but it's important to remember that this is only part of the equation. If you try to resolve body composition issues by just exercising more and more, you risk depleting essential nutrients such as magnesium, B vitamins and zinc. Exercise also increases the production of the stress hormones cortisol and adrenaline. Too much of these on a long-term basis may even increase fat storage! Extended periods of exercise will also raise appetite levels; not a great idea if you already struggle to keep your appetite under control.

In our role as personal trainers, we have also observed many people adopt a sense of dietary complacency as they increase their training routine. They consume more processed foods, alcohol and calories in general with a belief they could simply **"burn it off on Monday."** However, as mentioned earlier, these foods and habits (including exercise) in excess will all have greater physiological consequences and possibly compromise long-term health. Many studies support frequent daily walking and a couple of shorter, more intense exercise sessions to support hormonal communication. Take a moment to assess whether you've taken the 'exercise more' advice to another level and actually need to scale it back a little and invest more in your nutrition.

THE NATURAL SOLUTION

Ideally you don't want to be spending your life just counting calories and sweating it out for hours in the gym to maintain a healthy weight. Even if you have the willpower to do it, this is not what we consider to be optimal health. Life is a journey that should be full of wonderful experiences, and not just a mission to lose weight. **Excess body fat needs to be addressed by reviewing your energy intake, energy expenditure, eating behaviors, the source of your calories and lifestyle.**[64]

This is what we love most about paleo-ish nutrition: that you are naturally favoring unprocessed nutrition and therefore decreasing the hyperpalatability of your food, yet still making sure that it's incredibly tasty. Simply changing the source of your calories to more ancestral varieties encourages hormone sensitivity and feedback, supporting healthy weight regulation.

Remember that your health is a lifestyle, and that other factors, including sleep and stress, also make a contribution. So make sure you check out our Healthy Habits for Success on page 64.

CHAPTER 3
Grains, Gluten, Legumes & Dairy

In our first book we outlined some of the arguments for avoiding or limiting consumption of grains, legumes and some dairy products. While they are not necessarily an essential component of nutrition and you can source the nutrients they contain in other Fitter Foods, many people enjoy dishes that include them. Here we offer you some background information, guidance and tips to help you establish whether you wish to include them on a regular or occasional basis.

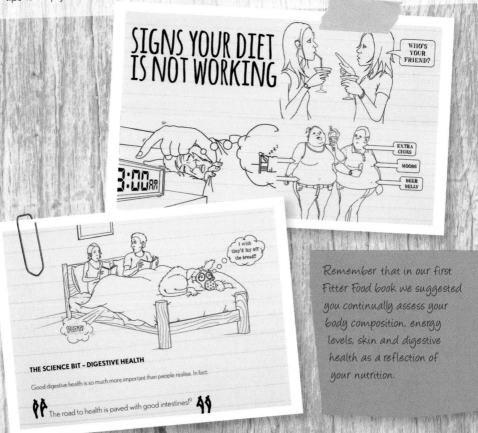

SIGNS YOUR DIET IS NOT WORKING

WHO'S YOUR FRIEND?

EXTRA CHINS

MOOBS

BEER BELLY

I wish they'd lay off the bread!!

POOT!

THE SCIENCE BIT – DIGESTIVE HEALTH

Good digestive health is so much more important than people realise. In fact,

The road to health is paved with good intestines!?

Remember that in our first Fitter Food book we suggested you continually assess your body composition, energy levels, skin and digestive health as a reflection of your nutrition.

MISSING YOUR MORNING OATMEAL?

We must have received over 100 emails about gluten-free oats, so we have gathered that many people must be missing oatmeal! What is most important in deciding your breakfast menu is that you make the right decision for you and personalize Paleo Primer to your own health history, macronutrient needs and the feedback you experience from your body after implementing any nutritional changes.

Research on the health effects of grains is still inconclusive, as good scientific studies are still lacking. One way to inform your choice is to consider some of the studies conducted for celiac suffers who have an immune response to gluten grains. For those who have experienced issues with grain-based foods before, plant classifications detailed below may be significant.

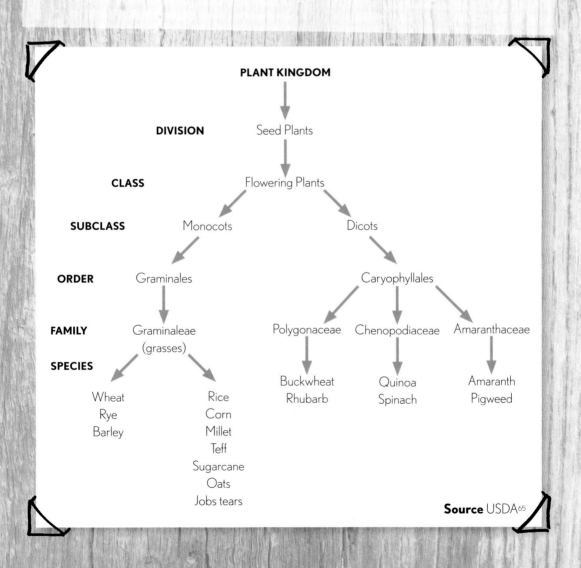

PLANT KINGDOM

DIVISION — Seed Plants

CLASS — Flowering Plants

SUBCLASS — Monocots / Dicots

ORDER — Graminales / Caryophyllales

FAMILY — Graminaleae (grasses) / Polygonaceae / Chenopodiaceae / Amaranthaceae

SPECIES

Wheat, Rye, Barley
Rice, Corn, Millet, Teff, Sugarcane, Oats, Jobs tears
Buckwheat, Rhubarb
Quinoa, Spinach
Amaranth, Pigweed

Source USDA[65]

29

Some types of grains are better tolerated and do not appear to trigger the same number of immune issues. The following summary by Donald Kasarda, Ph.D., for the USDA details the relevance of plant classifications:

★ Wheat, rye and barley are closely related as a tribe in the grass family under a plant classification called Hordeae or Triticeae. Spelt and kamut are also types of wheat. All of these have proteins shown to be toxic to celiac patients.

★ Oats are naturally gluten-free but are often contaminated with gluten as they are farmed and processed alongside wheat (unless labelled 'gluten-free'). Oats belong to a separate tribe of grasses. However, the proteins in oats known as avenins are similar in structure to wheat proteins, so those who cannot tolerate wheat may benefit from avoiding or limiting oat intake.

★ Rice and corn are part of the grass family, but the proteins do not seem to interact with the immune system in the same way and thus are usually better tolerated by celiacs. Millet, sorghum and teff are genetically very close to corn.

★ Dicotyledonous plants ("dicots") are only very distantly related to the grass family and include buckwheat, quinoa and amaranth. These are often referred to as "pseudo grains" and have their own subset of seed proteins, but studies up to this point suggest these are often better tolerated by celiacs.

QUICK GUIDE TO GRAINS

TIP
You can always pimp your grains with more nutrient-dense foods—use sourdough bread as a platform for butter and liver paté, or stir some egg yolks and cocoa into your oatmeal.

★ Grains offer very little nutrition in terms of vitamins and minerals, so if you have some health issues that you're looking to resolve, you may benefit from choosing more nutrient-dense foods and ancestral sources of carbohydrates.

★ If you have digestive or immune-related disorders, you will benefit from trialling a grain-free diet for 1-3 months and then reintroducing pseudo grains before experimenting with other grains.

★ If you have excess body fat, you may need to improve insulin health and benefit from limiting grain-based carbohydrates, instead favoring vegetables and sweet potatoes (see Chapter 5).

★ If you participate in intense exercise or endurance sports you may find that including grain-based foods is helpful to increase your carbohydrate intake (see Chapter 5). As exercise places an added stress on the digestive and immune system, you might benefit from choosing some minimally processed, gluten-free grains, including the pseudo grains, rice, oats and corn.

★ Artisan grain products prepared with more traditional methods (including sprouting and fermenting) and organic ingredients will likely have a greater nutrient content, and the longer preparation process will improve the digestibility of the grains (although they are still not advised for those with autoimmune problems). One of the most traditional methods of preparing bread is through long sourdough fermentation; ideally this is carried out over 12-24 hours.

THE GREAT GLUTEN DEBATE

Gluten-free diets have become rather fashionable these days, with a number of celebrities leading the movements. Sadly, this has led many people to jump on the band wagon with little to no understanding of the reasons behind or benefits of avoiding gluten, with others dismissing it as another fad diet. Some people genuinely need to be 100% gluten-free and experience significant health benefits from minimizing their exposure to gluten.

To help you fully understand and decide whether or not you should eliminate gluten from your nutrition, we refer you to gastroenterologist and researcher Dr. Alessio Fasano.[66] Dr. Fasano's research established that not only does celiac disease affect a much higher percentage of the population than previously suspected, but almost **one third of the US population has a genetic predisposition to celiac disease**. However, only a fraction of people with this predisposition fully develop the disease, so there are other environmental factors that may influence the onset of gluten-related health disorders.[67] His research also discovered that another reaction to gluten exists, now referred to as non-celiac gluten sensitivity. This suggests that there may be a spectrum of gluten-related disorders.[68]

In our first book and in Chapter 1 we emphasized the importance of digestive health, building up an army of healthy bacteria in your gut while keeping the lining of the gastrointestinal tract strong so that it can provide a protective barrier. The digestive system is essentially the outside world inside your body. Dr. Fasano discovered how the proteins in gluten lead to the production of a protein called zonulin. Zonulin causes the breakdown of the tight junctions between the cells that line the intestinal wall. If this happens continuously or to a large extent, it creates a scenario referred to as "leaky gut." This process plays a role in the development of celiac and other autoimmune diseases, including type 1 diabetes and some nervous system disorders.[69]

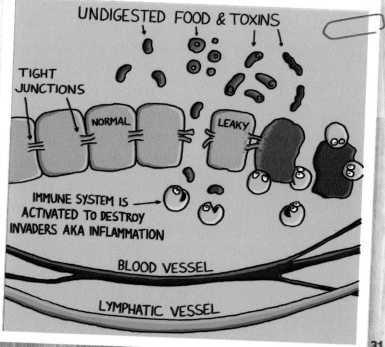

QUICK COACHING SESSION:
WHAT IS AN AUTOIMMUNE DISEASE?

An autoimmune disease is an illness that occurs when the immune system starts to attack the body's own tissues.

Our immune system is like a gangster movie with many different characters having unique roles yet all engaged in a complex plot to root out and destroy invaders in the body. The immune system is always trying to get ahead of the game and educate itself to anticipate any future threats. It keeps a trophy piece of each bacteria or virus for future reference and parades it around the body to inform the rest of the gang what the bad guys look like.

Sometimes this system goes a little wrong and members of our immune system start parading around samples of our own tissues. The heavies then go and attack our organs, muscle tissue or nervous system. Exactly where they attack determines the type of autoimmune disease.

Although gluten has been established as a trigger for celiac disease, it is believed there may be several environmental triggers, many yet to be identified. Leaky gut is always present in the development of autoimmune problems.

Chris Kresser[70] brilliantly summarizes the triggers of autoimmune problems as including "a modern Western diet, chronic stress, changes in the gut microbiome, environmental toxins, sleep deprivation, vitamin D deficiency, reduced sun exposure and ?"—as there are likely other factors yet to be identified.

TYPES OF AUTOIMMUNE DISEASE

★ Autoimmune hemolytic anemia
★ Pernicious anemia
★ Autoimmune thrombocytopenia
★ Antiphospholipid syndrome (APS)
★ Temporal artertis
★ Anti-phospholipid syndrome
★ Vasculitides such as Wegener's granulomatosis
★ Behcet's disease
★ Type 1 or immune mediated diabetes mellitus
★ Grave's Disease
★ Hashimoto's thyroiditis
★ Autoimmune oophoritis and orchitis
★ Autoimmune disease of the adrenal gland
★ Crohn's Disease
★ Ulcerative colitis
★ Primary biliary cirrhosis
★ Autoimmune hepatitis
★ Rheumatoid arthritis
★ Systemic lupus erythematosus
★ Scleroderma
★ Polymyositis, dermatomyositis
★ Spondyloarthropathies such as ankylosing spondylitis
★ Sjogren's syndrome
★ Multiple sclerosis
★ Myasthenia gravis
★ Autoimmune neuropathies such as Guillain-Barre
★ Autoimmune ureitis
★ Psoriasis
★ Dermatitis herpetiformis
★ Pemphigus vulgaris
★ Vitiligo

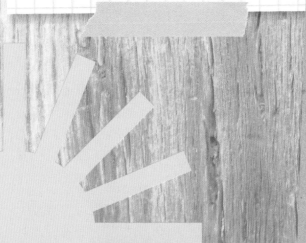

PALEO PRIMER AND AUTOIMMUNE PROBLEMS

In addition to following the Fitter Food principles of avoiding processed and refined foods, individuals with autoimmune conditions may also benefit from eliminating the following:

- ✔ Grains & pseudo grains (wheat, rice, amaranth, barley, oats, buckwheat, rye, corn, quinoa, spelt and millet)
- ✔ All dairy products (some people can tolerate ghee and butter)
- ✔ Nuts (almonds, cashews, hazelnuts, Brazil nuts, walnuts). Coconut and macadamias are sometimes fine.
- ✔ Legumes (lentils, chickpeas, peas, peanuts, soy beans, kidney beans and fava beans)
- ✔ Eggs (chicken, duck and goose)
- ✔ Nightshades (cayenne, chili pepper, eggplant, goji berry, peppers, paprika, potatoes, tomatoes)
- ✔ Seeds (anise, caraway, chia, cumin, coriander, fenugreek, mustard, nutmeg, poppy, pumpkin, sunflower, sesame and hemp)
- ✔ Alcohol
- ✔ Coffee
- ✔ Cocoa (carob can be used as a substitute)

It's wise to trial this approach for 1–3 months, depending upon your results and then experiment with adding foods back into your nutrition carefully.

REINTRODUCING FOODS

When reintroducing foods back into your diet it's important to do so slowly, with some careful structure and monitoring to assess whether a food item acts as a trigger for any health symptoms you experience.

The following may be a sign of a possible reaction:
- ★ Gas or bloating
- ★ Constipation, sluggish or uncomfortable bowel movements
- ★ Loose and frequent bowel movements (>3 times a day)
- ★ Skin issues: rashes, acne, itchy skin
- ★ Muscle or joint pains or aches
- ★ Depression, fatigue or a foggy head

TIPS
- ✔ Introduce 1 food or drink item at a time, **NOT** an entire food group. For example, butter (not all dairy products) or green tea (not all caffeinated beverages).
- ✔ Use a food diary as shown on page 46 to monitor your responses.
- ✔ Allow 2–3 days to assess the results before any further reintroductions.

REINTRODUCTION
When reintroducing foods, begin with those that offer the most nutrition first of all:
- ★ Egg yolks, then whole eggs
- ★ Butter or ghee
- ★ Fermented dairy (yogurt, kefir)
- ★ Nightshade vegetables

Finally test out 'optional foods', including grains, legumes, caffeinated beverages, alcohol, nuts, sweeteners and cocoa.

See Chris Kresser's *The Paleo Cure* (www.paleocurebook.com) for a more in-depth, step-by-step guide to reintroducing food.

TO GLUTEN OR NOT TO GLUTEN...
YOU DECIDE!

If you consider that we only started farming crops containing gluten a few thousand years ago, gluten grains are a late addition to the human diet, and perhaps we don't fully understand the implications of this nutritional transition.

Celiac disease, gluten sensitivity and wheat allergies all present a convincing argument for avoiding, or at the very least limiting, gluten consumption. We certainly **DO NOT NEED** these foods in our nutrition. However, it's equally important to remember that not everyone develops health issues, despite long-term consumption. For some people the occasional pizza, piece of bread or bottle of beer will not present any major health complications. In fact there are times it might just be good for the soul. ☺

Here is a little round up of the facts so you can decide where you wish stand in **THE GREAT GLUTEN DEBATE**.

1 Given the association between gluten and autoimmune conditions, it is advisable to avoid gluten 100% if you suffer from any autoimmune disease listed on page 32.

2 If you are genetically predisposed to autoimmune conditions and they exist within your immediate family, you will likely benefit from significantly limiting your consumption of gluten-containing foods and should consider total elimination to minimize the risk of autoimmune problems in the future.

3 It is believed that the onset of an autoimmune disease is influenced by other factors, including chronic stress, vitamin D deficiency, sleep deprivation and environmental toxins. If you frequently experience any of these, you should ideally address them. However, if these are unmodifiable lifestyle factors, for example, if you work night shifts, then you will likely benefit by optimizing your nutrition and limiting gluten.

4 To really assess the impact of a gluten-free diet, why not run a short trial on yourself? Studies have observed that trialling a gluten-free diet can improve irritable bowel syndrome[71] and other health conditions, including autism[72] and epilepsy.[73] If you are experiencing health issues, try eliminating gluten for three months to fully assess the potential benefit it may bring.

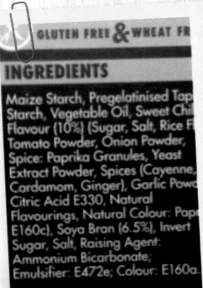

GLUTEN FREE & WHEAT FR

INGREDIENTS

Maize Starch, Pregelatinised Tap
Starch, Vegetable Oil, Sweet Chil
Flavour (10%) (Sugar, Salt, Rice Fl
Tomato Powder, Onion Powder,
Spice: Paprika Granules, Yeast
Extract Powder, Spices (Cayenne,
Cardamom, Ginger), Garlic Powd
Citric Acid E330, Natural
Flavourings, Natural Colour: Papr
E160c), Soya Bran (6.5%), Invert
Sugar, Salt, Raising Agent:
Ammonium Bicarbonate;
Emulsifier: E472e; Colour: E160a.

GLUTEN-FREE FOODS

If you wish to avoid gluten 100%, you might wish to use some gluten-free flours for things like baking. However, be cautious of packaged gluten-free products. Check the labels and you will see they contain a number of unrecognizable ingredients. In fact, some are more junk food than real food, so keep these on the occasional list.

WANT SOME BEANS ON YOUR SOURDOUGH TOAST?

Excitingly, some recent evidence suggests that Neanderthal man loved beans on toast. Well, OK to be more accurate, he may have enjoyed eating legumes and properly prepared grains.[74] The case with legumes is very similar to grains in that if you have health issues to resolve, you should focus more on the foundation foods in the Fitter Food pyramid. Also, if you have any digestive disorders, legumes are a little notorious for their fart factor, especially if not prepared properly. This involves soaking and cooking the beans for long periods of time. If you're clearing the room with your bottom burps, consider avoiding legumes and revisit our guidance on page 12 to improve healthy gut function before reintroducing.

One of the best ways to consume legumes is to cook them yourself from scratch. If using canned varieties, try to avoid preservatives and rinse them throughly. All legumes, with the exception of split peas and lentils, should be soaked prior to cooking to improve digestibility and decrease cooking time. If consuming these on a regular basis a pressure cooker is a worthwhile investment. Here's a quick reference guide:

LEGUME PREPARATION & COOKING CHART

DRIED BEANS 1 CUP	SOAKING TIME	COOKING TIME	PRESSURE COOKING TIME
Adzuki Beans	None	45-50 mins	15-20 mins
Black Beans	Overnight	45-60 mins	15-20 mins
Black Eyed Peas	Overnight	1 hour	10 mins
Chick Peas	Overnight	1 ½-2 ½ hours	15-20 mins
Kidney Beans	Overnight	1-1 ½ hours	10 mins
Lentils, Green	None	30-45 mins	6-8 mins
Lentils, Red	None	20-30 mins	5-7 mins
Lima Beans	Overnight	60-90 mins	Not recommended
Mung Beans	Overnight	1-1 ½ hours	8-10 mins
Navy Beans	Overnight	45-60 mins	4-5 mins
Peas, Split	None	35-40 mins	Not recommended
Pinto Beans	Overnight	1-1 ½ hours	10 mins

DO YOU DO DAIRY?

Dairy is a nutrient-dense group of foods, especially if sourced from farmers who raise the animals in their natural environment, feed them on grass and care for their welfare. All dairy offers a range of micronutrients and healthy fats.[75] However, grass-fed dairy produce invariably has greater amounts.[76]

Some people have allergies or sensitivities to the proteins in dairy, either whey or casein (or both). They are often unable to digest these proteins properly, which means the proteins damage the intestinal cells and potentially trigger an immune reaction. This is particularly common among individuals who have a gluten sensitivity as milk proteins commonly cross-react with gluten.[77]

A number of people also suffer from lactose intolerance, where the sugar in dairy products causes digestive issues. Lactose intolerance can be due to a number of factors. These include not having enough beneficial bacteria, which play a role in the breakdown and digestion of lactose. Or the intestinal cells may be damaged; these are responsible for producing lactase, the digestive enzyme that breaks down lactose.

Certain populations also stop producing lactase enzymes during childhood. Some researchers suggested that perhaps we shouldn't be consuming milk products after this age; however, recent studies have shown this may be more genetically predetermined as cultures that traditionally consume milk are more likely to continue producing lactase enzymes into adulthood. This is known as lactase persistence.[78]

Many people also enjoy dairy products and want to make them a regular feature of their nutrition. However, if you have health symptoms and wish to determine if these are food related, the best means of assessing whether dairy is implicated is to eliminate all dairy products for 30 days and then reintroduce them slowly, using the steps outlined on page 33 to monitor the results. When you reintroduce dairy products, use the following diagram as a guide and begin with high-fat dairy products first, as these will contain the lowest levels of lactose and protein.

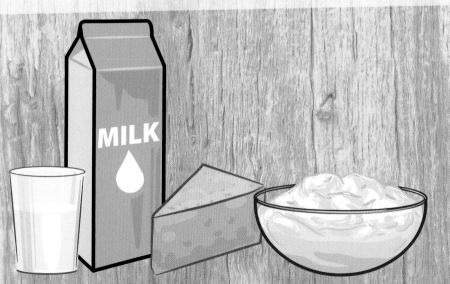

**LOW LACTOSE
HIGH FAT
LOW PROTEIN CONTENT**

START HERE AS THESE ARE MORE LIKELY TO BE TOLERATED, AND WORK YOUR WAY DOWN.

★ **GHEE:** butter boiled to remove the milk solids

★ **BUTTER:** contains predominantly fat and <1% lactose

★ **FERMENTED MILK (KEFIR) OR YOGURT:** ideally this should be homemade or unpasteurized/raw. The bacteria consume the lactose sugar, lowering the content.

★ **ICE CREAM:** Matt's favorite ☺ contains 3.1–8.4% lactose.

★ **DOUBLE CREAM:** contains predominantly fat and around 2.8–3.0% lactose.

★ **CHEESE:** the amount of lactose is generally low, but will vary across types. Some hard cheeses are very low BUT higher in casein protein.

★ **MILK:** contains 3.7–5.1% lactose. Skimmed and semi-skimmed have a higher lactose content than whole milk.

**HIGHER LACTOSE
HIGHER PROTEIN CONTENT**

HANDY TIPS

★ If you experience digestive issues after drinking milk, including bloating, gas or indigestion, you may be suffering from intolerance to the A1 protein found in most cows' milk. In this case, some recent research suggests that A2 varieties of cows' milk could be better tolerated.[79] You might also wish to experiment with sheep, goat and buffalo dairy products.

★ Studies have shown that probiotic supplementation, along with consumption of small amounts of live yogurt, can support lactose tolerance by improving the balance and activity of the gut bacteria.[80]

★ Eating prebiotic foods including garlic, leeks, artichokes and onions can also improve the digestion of dairy by increasing levels of the bacteria that produce lactase enzymes.

★ Raw dairy produce has not undergone pasteurization, and so it retains many of the enzymes and bacteria that support the digestion of lactose. Many people find they can tolerate this form of dairy better than pasteurized.

WHICH WHEY WILL YOU GO?

Whey is the liquid by-product of cheese-making, but is more probably known to you as a sports or weight-loss supplement. Many people take protein supplements with little understanding of the role they can play within nutrition or the potential benefits they have to offer, so here's a short guide to help you out.

REMEMBER

If you can't tolerate whey protein, you can use vegetarian protein powders as a supplement to your nutrition including rice, hemp and pea protein. See page 73 for our recommendations.

BENEFITS OF WHEY

- Whey is often preferred as a protein supplement due to its high bioavailability; it is quickly digested and absorbed.[81]
- Whey has been shown to support immune health by increasing levels of glutathione, the master antioxidant in the body.[82]
- Whey is currently being explored for its potential anti-cancer properties.[83]
- Whey protein can positively enhance immune function by improving antimicrobial activity.[84]
- Whey protein provides a rich source of branch chain amino acids and L-glutamine which help to retain muscle mass and aid recovery.[85][86]
- Whey can support weight loss and improve satiety.[87]

WHEY CONCENTRATE VS. WHEY PROTEIN ISOLATE

There are numerous debates about which is the better option. However, it's really based upon your own personal preference. If you're training frequently and wish to use a protein supplement for convenience and to support performance goals, consider your digestive health first in making a decision. Whey protein isolate is subjected to some additional manufacturing processes which yield a higher protein, lower lactose and lower fat content, so it's usually the best option for lactose intolerance.[88] There is an added price tag when sourcing a good quality brand and isolate is often more expensive, so your budget may feature in your final choice. As with other dairy products, grass-fed is the best.

CHAPTER 3
HEALTHY TAKEAWAYS

If you have health issues you wish to resolve, you will likely improve these by focusing on nutrient density and mainly eating the foundation foods in the Fitter Food pyramid. If you have a history of digestive or autoimmune disorders, a grain and legume-free diet will often be a beneficial choice. However, if all is good in the hood and you want to vary your nutritional intake, feel free to experiment.

CHAPTER 4
The Fitter Food Journey

If you've been eating cereal for breakfast, sandwiches for lunch and sticking a frozen dinner in the microwave for dinner, we totally understand that the thought of ditching these might seem a little daunting—or even impossible just now. We live in a world where convenience overrides health as a priority, and the notion of sourcing and cooking all of your own food might just be making you want to just close this book. Don't panic and definitely don't close the book! We have four simple steps you can implement straight away that will begin to transform your health but not drastically change your regular routine.

The key to starting out is to not over-think or rush the process. Step-by-step changes might be a better option for you. There's no race to implement all of our guidelines because there's no finish line. The changes you're adopting here should be considered lifelong, and there should be no need to return to the way you ate before. Fitter Food involves adopting a different mindset and lifestyle, and ultimately building a better body.

STEP 1: CHANGE BREAKFAST

We're big fans of eating a breakfast that contains healthy fats and protein in place of the carbohydrate-rich cereal, pastries and toast that most people consider to be breakfast options. A better balance of macronutrients is important in order to stabilize your blood sugar levels. This is especially important first thing in the morning, as it influences your energy, appetite and the cravings you may experience for the rest of the day. Healthy fats and protein also form the building blocks of the hormones that get us out of bed and help us to function optimally. Quick, easy options include:

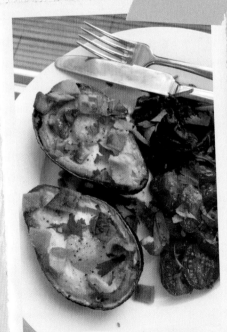

1 Poached eggs, smoked salmon, avocado and fruit
2 A protein smoothie (see pages 102-107)
3 Salty Banana Cinnamon Scramble (page 98)

KERIS'S FAVORITE BREAKFAST ☺

STEP 2: MAKE SIMPLE CARBOHYDRATE SWAPS

This move alone will deliver astounding health benefits by supporting optimal gut health and hormone signalling. All you need to do is ditch the bread, pasta, couscous, dinner rolls and crackers for root vegetables, white potatoes, sweet potatoes or fruit. All you're doing here is replacing a carbohydrate for a carbohydrate but opting for single-ingredient, unprocessed foods. When transitioning away from processed foods, don't change your macronutrient ratios too much initially; just change the source.

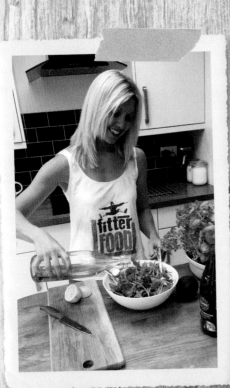

STEP 3: GET SOME KITCHEN TRAINING SESSIONS IN

To really make or break your Fitter Food experience— you're going to need to become a savvy chef. This involves getting back into the kitchen for a few culinary training sessions. Luckily we're not chefs, so all our recipes are **DEAD EASY**, with minimal ingredients and steps. When cooking your own food you can always ensure it's full of nothing but awesome, fresh ingredients and in no time at all you'll become incredibly proud of the tasty creations you've made. In fact, one of the great things about becoming a Fitter Foodie is the enthusiasm you will develop for quality ingredients and kitchen equipment.

STEP 4: AIM FOR AN 80:20 APPROACH

One thing that often puts people off making changes to their nutrition is the idea of giving up their favorite foods. However, this needn't be the case. You don't necessarily need to start out 100%, especially if you know the pressure will cause you to fall off the wagon. Some people succeed much better with a more relaxed attitude, implementing one step at a time. This may feel more sustainable and will ensure that your progress continues. Start by changing breakfast and then work towards ensuring that 80% of your meals are based on Fitter Food principles. Once you've done that, we're pretty sure you'll experience amazing results.

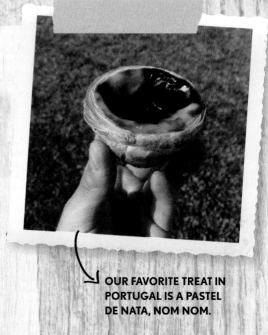

OUR FAVORITE TREAT IN PORTUGAL IS A PASTEL DE NATA, NOM NOM.

DON'T BE A CARRIED-AWAY CAVEMAN

On the other hand, you may have been dabbling with your nutrition for some time and perhaps feel a little overwhelmed with all the tasks and information on the table. In this case it might be wise for you to step away a little and put things back into perspective.

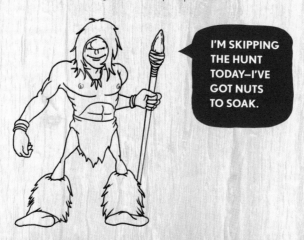

I'M SKIPPING THE HUNT TODAY—I'VE GOT NUTS TO SOAK.

We can even take some guidance from our ancestors here. If they discovered a new form of sustenance they would have a nibble to test it out. If it made them sick or ill they might try preparing it in a different way: soaking, cooking, fermenting or drying before trying to eat it again. If it still made them sick they didn't eat it—simple. If a food or drink item tasted good and there was no negative reaction they knew it was safe to continue eating—simple!

What might start out as a straightforward desire for self-improvement can sometimes develop into an obsession and a relentless mission to super optimize every mouthful you eat. With a search engine at your fingertips 24/7, maintaining your nutrition can easily become a full-time job, and it's easy to invest hours researching countless, often unnecessary details.

Falling into this pattern of behavior means that life itself can be placed on hold, because you can't risk any social situation where gluten might be present, or you're left with little time for wonderful experiences with friends and family because cabbage needs to be fermented. Ironically, overwhelming yourself in this way is more likely to have a negative impact on your natural, instinctive relationship with your food.

The stress of striving for the perfect plate may actually do you more harm than good.

THIS IS ROB, THE EDITOR OF OUR FITTER FOOD RADIO PODCAST, BONDING WITH MATT OVER A SHARED LOVE OF ICE CREAM

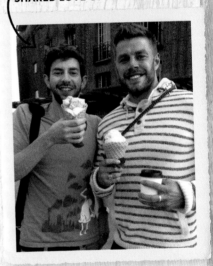

This situation easily occurs because many of us experience a range of benefits when we transition back towards ancestral nutrition. While there may be some things you absolutely need to eliminate on a long-term basis, there are many steps on the path to feeling more awesome. So if a waiter accidently serves your salad with a sprinkling of croutons, it needn't elicit a full panic attack.

It's important to remember that nutrition is just one aspect of your health. It provides a source of fuel and while it's important to meet your body's needs, human cultures have always gone to considerable lengths to obtain food and drink items they desire and enjoy. Not all choices should be governed by your health needs alone.

Nutrition also has significance beyond sustenance. It's an important gift your mother gives you from her own body from the moment you are conceived. It's an experience we share with friends and family. It brings communities together to celebrate and socialize. It's an expression of true generosity; we love nothing more than laying out a feast of deliciousness for our loved ones.

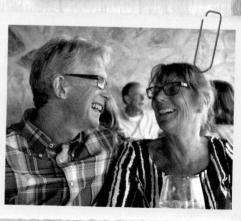

Food embodies love, friendships, relationships and forms part of some amazing life experiences; never forget that in your quest for health. BOSH!

EXPERT ADVICE FROM FITTER FRIENDS

During our own journey, we've met some awesome characters and been inspired by their passion, dedication and common-sense yet holistic approach to health and nutrition. We asked each of them to share with you their personal perceptions regarding optimal health.

DR. TOMMY WOOD
A Primal Doctor's Perspective

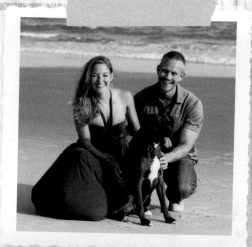

There is a huge amount of easily-accessible and contradictory information available about diet and lifestyle nowadays. Though sometimes it doesn't seem like it, everybody out there discussing health has important knowledge to offer, and most of us genuinely want to help others. But instead of discussing these things, we engage in battles over our information because we are certain that others are wrong. This happens because we like to form groups, and we like to be right. But what if it's not that simple? Paleo. Veganism. Low-carb. Calorie counting. I think it's important to remember that all of these ideas have data and first-hand experience that can back them up. However, anybody that sits firmly in any one of these groups has also misinterpreted (or ignored) data that disagrees with their viewpoint. For me, the simplest way to describe how to work towards optimal health is to do the things we did regularly over the last couple of million years of evolution. Sleep. Get outdoors. Move. Eat enough food. Have sex. Minimize chronic stressors. All of that will help you achieve your goals. But remember that worrying about doing everything perfectly also counts as a chronic stressor. Yes, certain food groups should be avoided for certain people, but removing processed foods and learning to cook and move will get most people most of the way.

As we look at the bigger picture, I truly believe that you can integrate all the seemingly disparate ideas about health, and use basic human physiology, biochemistry and genetics to show why one group being right doesn't necessarily make another group wrong. Even better, the real upshot of all the conflicting advice is that we all get to figure out what works for us and makes us feel and perform best! Just remember that it's okay to be wrong, and it's okay to make mistakes. And sometimes, or maybe more than sometimes, it's okay to eat a lot of ice cream.

HEALTH AND FITNESS IN THE REAL WORLD
WWW.DRRAGNAR.COM

43

EMMA MIHILL
A Naturopath's Perspective

When you first become interested in your health and you begin to unravel a whole crazy mess of information, it's very easy to become completely overwhelmed with the contradictory–yet plausible–advice available from every expert under the sun. My journey into nutrition came from wanting to find the optimal diet so I could feel the best I possibly could. Over the years my approach has stemmed from following various strict regimes, and although these may have had reasonable applications I could identify with, I have discovered that the real science and the real research comes from you, an individual, with your own individual needs, and not from anything I would call 'pure science.' Years of self-experimenting and education and just LIVING have finally left me content and happy, knowing that the answer is quite simply this: If it has grown/lived on earth or grown/lived in the sea, you're probably on the right path!

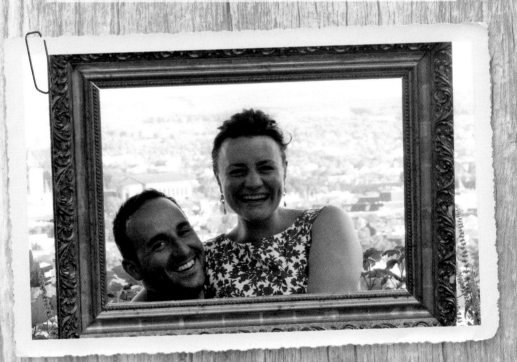

RANNOCH DONALD
Movement Maverick & Founder of the 100 Rep Challenge

We are what we repeatedly do. Habits, good and bad, occupy the same space. To positively impact our health and fitness we need to make conscious decisions about the food we eat, the way we move and how we recover. Excellence is a habit…

And consistency is key. The 100 Rep Challenge grew out of a desire to provide people with ways to engage in everyday activity. By providing a simple framework, from walking to body weight training, with a focus on simple drills, minimal equipment and skilful movement, the 100 Rep Challenge has encouraged thousands of people to get a little more movement in their day while removing the guesswork.

We run 100 Rep Challenges at gyms, clubs and fitness expos but the real challenge is a personal one. Irrespective of age, ability or gender, we encourage individuals to master the basics of body weight training, set personal challenges, develop skill and strength and, in turn, use that experience to inspire others to do the same. With the 100 Rep Challenge, everyone is a coach and we are all role models (yes, YOU!), whether we realize it or not.

Vitamin EDA (Every Day Activity):
Side effects may include, improved mood,
lower blood pressure, fat loss,
improved cognition, improved strength
and joint health, reduced stress,
better sexual function, better sleep.

In the words of Arthur Ashe,
"Start where you are, use what you have,
do what you can."

WWW.100REPCHALLENGE.COM

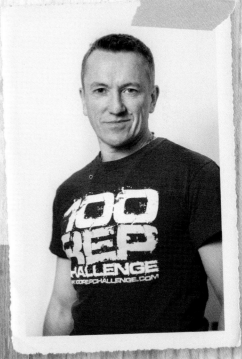

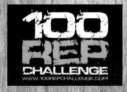

CHAPTER 5
Personalizing Your Fitter Food

We're all unique little snowflakes when it comes to nutrition. We have our own gene profile, balance of hormones, mental wellbeing, balance of gut bacteria, environment, lifestyle and routine. While everyone can benefit from Fitter Food principles, there's no one size fits all, and sometimes you may need to explore the finer details. The following tools provide some guidance on how to establish your own nutrient needs and adapt your nutritional intake accordingly.

ASSESS YOUR FITTER FEEDBACK

In the last few chapters, we have mentioned implementing changes to your nutrition and lifestyle and continually assessing the feedback your body offers. There are different methods you can use to track the results you experience. The following are a couple of options:

1. Keep a food, lifestyle and symptom diary.

Record your daily food and drink intake. Note the time it was consumed and how it made you feel. You can also add lifestyle details, including how much sleep you had the night before, how much exercise you performed that day and your current stress levels. You can also use this to track improvements to any health symptoms, including bloating or skin issues.

fitter

FOOD AND LIFESTYLE DIARY

TIME	MEAL	FOOD/FLUID/ SUPPLEMENT INTAKE	REACTIONS		
			BEFORE	IMMEDIATELY AFTER	2 HOURS AFTER
	BREAKFAST				
	SNACK				
	LUNCH				
	SNACK				
	DINNER				
	EVENING SNACK				
	TRAINING				
HOURS OF SLEEP			MINDFUL ACTIVITY		

WEB: www.fitterfood.com   **EMAIL:** info@fitterfood.com   **FACEBOOK:** Facebook.com/FitterFood   **TWITTER:** @fitter_food

2. Take photos and measurements.

This method of assessing your body composition is preferable to using weighing scales as many people have an intimate history with their weight and attach emotional significance to the numbers on the scales. This often causes a great deal of anxiety and stress. Weighing yourself is also often highly inaccurate as a method of assessing fat loss, because your weight is influenced by other factors, including muscle mass and your hydration levels. The scales will also fluctuate across the day and week, and for ladies the menstrual cycle will influence the reading. In fact, you may even notice that the numbers on the scales increase as your body converts fat to lean muscle, especially if you are participating in resistance exercise. **FYI, THIS IS A GOOD THING!** Your resting metabolism will be higher, your insulin sensitivity will be greater and you're burning fat... **WHOOP!**

You can use the following as an alternative:

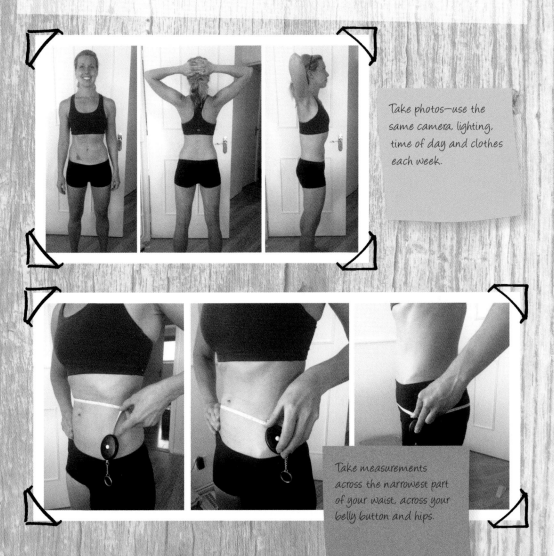

Take photos—use the same camera, lighting, time of day and clothes each week.

Take measurements across the narrowest part of your waist, across your belly button and hips.

3. Assess calorie intake.

In the last few decades there has been far too much emphasis on calorie counting as the ultimate weight loss solution. If you rely solely on this as a means of losing body fat you're unlikely to be able to maintain the results. That being said, it can be a useful tool if adopted sensibly along with some key changes to the source of your calories and in your lifestyle habits.

CALCULATE YOUR CALORIE NEEDS

Calculating your calorie needs allows you to establish your energy requirements for the day. The first step involves calculating your Basal Metabolic Rate (BMR). This is based upon your age, weight and height and is an estimate of the basic caloric need for your body to perform essential biological processes including breathing, digestion and cardiovascular function. It does not take into account any physical activity.

The Mifflin St. Jeor equation is one of the more accurate methods.[89] You can calculate your BMR at **www.bmi-calculator.net/bmr-calculator/**

Once you have established your basic calorie needs, you need to factor in your daily physical activity level. This can be done using the Harris Benedict Formula:

HARRIS BENEDICT FORMULA

★ **Little/no exercise:** BMR x 1.2 = Total Calorie Need
★ **Light exercise (1–3 days per week):** BMR x 1.375 = Total Calorie Need
★ **Moderate exercise (3–5 days/wk):** BMR x 1.55 = Total Calorie Need
★ **Very active (6-7 days/wk):** BMR x 1.725 = Total Calorie Need
★ **Extra active (very active & physical job):** BMR x 1.9 = Total Calorie Need

MY FITNESS PAL

My Fitness Pal (www.myfitnesspal.com) is a free calorie counting app that is available on iOS and Android devices as well as the Web. You can use it to calculate your BMR and calorie needs, factoring in your physical activity levels. Then input your nutritional intake for a few weeks to gain an insight into your energy balance, including total calories consumed, calorie expenditure and how much fat, protein and carbohydrates you consume.

IMPORTANT

Remember that food and drink items each elicit a hormonal response, so these calorie equations do NOT offer all the necessary information. They are just one small tool in your box.

INTERPRETING THE RESULTS

In the past it was suggested that simply eating less calories than you expended would result in fat loss. However, the human body is a little more complex than this simple formula would suggest. When we restrict calorie intake, several hormonal changes take place to compensate for the lack of nutrients and energy, including a decrease in your basal metabolic rate. Revisit the information on page 26 for a better understanding of this.

CALORIE STRATEGIES TO TRY

One approach you can take is to implement a small calorie deficit (consuming slightly less than your calorie needs). This won't bring about any drastic, negative hormonal changes or leave you with chronic hunger. Assess the impact for 2-4 weeks before making further changes. After this you may wish to try adjusting your intake by 5 or 10% to see if it has a positive impact.

Alternatively, if the results of your calorie review show that you've been in calorie deficit for a considerable period of time yet your body composition is static, it may be an indication that your body's metabolic rate has slowed down to conserve calories and is storing fat to protect you from starvation. Increasing your calorie intake incrementally may be more helpful in this case. We often see people who have cut their calories for a long time finally lose weight once they start eating more!

Use the calorie flowchart below to assess your calorie needs on an ongoing basis:

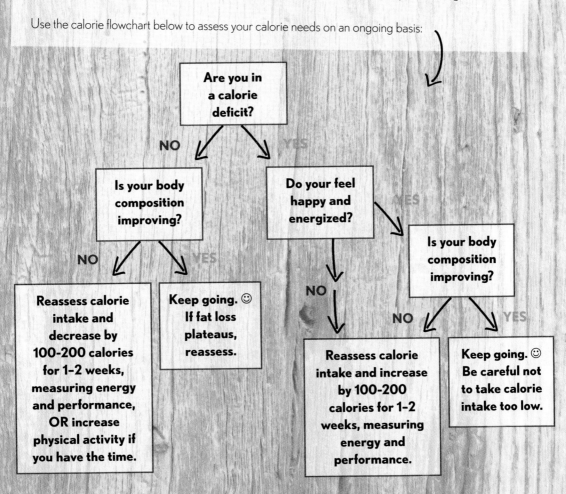

Are you in a calorie deficit?

NO → **Is your body composition improving?**

YES → **Do your feel happy and energized?**

Is your body composition improving? (NO)

NO → **Reassess calorie intake and decrease by 100-200 calories for 1–2 weeks, measuring energy and performance, OR increase physical activity if you have the time.**

YES → **Keep going. ☺ If fat loss plateaus, reassess.**

YES → **Is your body composition improving?**

NO → **Reassess calorie intake and increase by 100-200 calories for 1–2 weeks, measuring energy and performance.**

NO → **Reassess calorie intake and increase by 100-200 calories for 1–2 weeks, measuring energy and performance.**

YES → **Keep going. ☺ Be careful not to take calorie intake too low.**

ADAPTING MACRONUTRIENTS

In Chapter 2, we discussed the relevance of macronutrient intake. Remember that each has a different number of calories per gram:

★ Carb: 4 cals per gram
★ Protein: 4 cals per gram
★ Fat: 9 cals per gram
★ Alcohol: 7 cals per gram

**REMINDER FROM
CHAPTER 2**

Our bodies need macronutrients for energy. However, several factors can influence how we respond to different ratios and determine whether we feel better eating a high-fat diet or a high-carbohydrate diet. These include your genetic disposition, hormone health, digestive wellbeing and lifestyle factors including stress, exercise levels, sleep health and even the environment in which you live.

The studies of modern day hunter-gatherer tribes discussed in Chapter 2 observed radically different macronutrient intakes yet discovered that their chronic disease risks were low and their indicators of good health were far superior when compared to westernised societies. The most widely-studied are the Maasai and Kitavan tribes. The Maasai tribes from Kenya and Tanzania live primarily on milk from their cattle and consume around 70% of their calories from saturated fat. The Kitavan tribe, you may remember, are estimated to consume around 70% of their calories from carbohydrates, predominantly fruit, yams, sweet potato and taro. It's also important to point out that Western foods contribute almost nothing to their daily diets.

**THERE IS NO MAGICAL
MACRO FORMULA!**[90,91]

70% carbohydrates
& healthy

70% saturated fat
& healthy

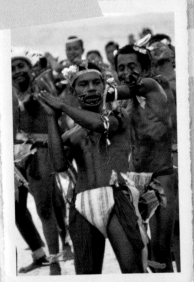

KITAVAN TRIBE

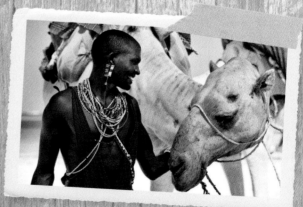

MASAI TRIBE

ESTABLISHING YOUR PROTEIN GOAL

Dietary proteins are an important part of balanced nutrition. The human body is unable to synthesise numerous amino acids, so they must be obtained from food. Many of the protein-rich foods we recommend such, as meat, fish, eggs and nuts are also good sources of vitamins or minerals. Our body is pretty much made out of protein, so it's hugely important to meet your requirements. Most people are aware that we need protein to retain and build lean muscle mass; however, every tissue in the body requires protein, including skin, hair, nails, bones and joints. It's also essential for most physiological functions, including hormonal communication and immune system health. The following table and working formula provide a guide to helping you establish your own intake and needs:

WORKING EXAMPLE
Female participating in 4 strength sessions a week.
Starting point = .82g protein per pound of bodyweight
Body weight = 143 pounds
143 lbs x .82g = 117g of protein daily

Remember this is grams of actual protein, not grams of fish or meat. To see what 117g of protein looks like, check out our quick reference guide on page 52.

MINIMUM PROTEIN GUIDELINES

TRAINING	PROTEIN (G/LB)
Frequent strength training and aiming to build muscle mass	.82g
Frequent endurance exercise	.68g
Sedentary	.54g

QUICK PROTEIN REFERENCE GUIDE

Just like our recipes, we like to keep this macro business simple. So here's a quick reference guide to help you hit your protein target without having to weigh your meals or make things complicated.

PROTEIN SOURCE	PORTION SIZE *Approximate weight*	PROTEIN CONTENT *Approximate values*
★ Bacon	2 slices / 38g	11g
★ Beef	Ground (20% fat) / 100g	19g
★ Burger	1 patty / 100g	20g
★ Cod	1 fillet / 140g	25g
★ Chicken breast	1 fillet / 125g	28g
★ Chicken drumstick	2 drumsticks / 200g	36.6g
★ Chicken thigh	3 thighs / 100g	19g
★ Cottage cheese	3 tbsp / 60g	6g
★ Eggs	1 medium	6g
★ Ham	1 slice / (24g)	5g
★ Lamb chop	2 chops / 55g	15g
★ Lamb	1 steak / 100g	29g
★ Lamb	Ground (20% fat) / 100g	17g
★ 20 nuts	28g	6-8g
★ Nut butter	1 tbsp	7-8g
★ Pork chop	85g	17g
★ Salmon	1 fillet / 100g	25g
★ Salmon	1 can / 213g	40g
★ Sardines	1 can / 120g	18g
★ Pork sausage	2 sausages / 60g	15g
★ Sea bass	1 fillet / 72g	16g
★ Shrimp	100g	14g
★ Steak fillet	155g	43g
★ Tuna	1 can / 160g	27g
★ Tuna	1 steak / 140g	35g
★ Turkey	Breast 1 slice / 28g	8g
★ Turkey	Ground breast / 100g	34g
★ Yogurt (Greek)	100g	7g

CARBOHYDRATE INTAKE

Carbohydrates provide a source of energy to the body. Once consumed, they are broken down into single molecules of sugar including glucose, fructose and galactose. Carbohydrates have acquired a bad reputation over the last few decades with the popularity of high-fat and high-protein diets, yet they make a perfectly healthy contribution to your nutrition. In fact, glucose is essential to a number of physiological functions. It is the preferred source of fuel for certain cells in our brain, as well as our red blood cells, and is required for healthy thyroid hormone function.

The human body can operate on a zero carbohydrate diet by converting protein or the backbone of fat molecules (triglycerides) into glucose, a process known as "gluconeogenesis." Many health researchers suggest the fact that the body goes to such great lengths to obtain glucose would suggest that we are well-adapted for carbohydrate consumption.

Carbohydrates should certainly not be vilified or blamed for body composition issues. However, our modern lifestyles do have a tendency to sabotage our ability to utilize carbohydrates effectively, leaving them to become stored as fats. The main nutrition and lifestyle factors that cause this include:

★ Processed and refined foods
★ Excess alcohol (more than two small servings)
★ Sedentary lifestyle
★ Over-exercising

★ Chronic stress
★ Excess caffeine
★ Excess refined sugar
★ Liquid calories (soft drinks, fruit juices)

Carrying excess body fat can be a sign that you have a compromised ability to metabolise glucose and that your cells are not using the carbohydrates you consume effectively. In this case you need to improve the lines of communication in the body and encourage cells to listen to the hormone insulin when it shouts out instructions to vacuum up the glucose from the blood stream so it can be used for various cellular functions. This is referred to as **"insulin sensitivity."**

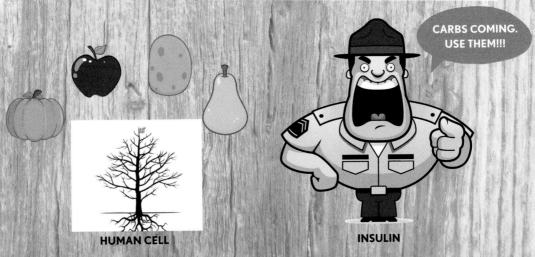

CARBS COMING. USE THEM!!!

HUMAN CELL

INSULIN

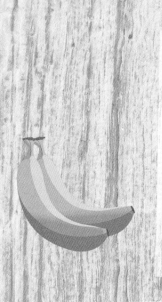

The following can all help improve insulin sensitivity:

- ✔ Frequent daily movement and walking. Aim for 10,000 steps daily.
- ✔ High intensity interval training 2-3 times a week
- ✔ Resistance training
- ✔ 8-9 hours of good quality sleep on a regular basis
- ✔ Herbs and spices
- ✔ Organ meats (a rich source of minerals that support insulin health)
- ✔ Magnesium-rich foods (spinach, dark chocolate, nuts)
- ✔ Limiting carbohydrates to vegetables and low-sugar fruits
- ✔ Managing stress
- ✔ Limiting caffeine and alcohol consumption

CARBOHYDRATE TIMING

As a minimum, we suggest you consume at least one fist-sized serving of starch-based carbohydrates (e.g. root vegetables, potatoes or rice) on a daily basis. In Chapter 2 we mentioned that studies have shown that consuming carbohydrates in the evening can help support a more optimal hormone profile during the day, regulating appetite and energy levels and even acting as a sleep aid at night.[92] Anecdotally many of our clients and Fitter 365 members have reported benefitting from this simple approach to carbohydrate consumption.

It's wise to consume carbohydrates after exercise as they will be used to refuel the body, replenish the glycogen used during exercise and support muscle preservation and recovery. If you also consume a little fruit post-exercise, the fructose (the sugar found in fruit) will be used to restore liver glycogen.

This also means that if you exercise first thing in the morning, you may prefer to consume the majority of your carbohydrates at breakfast. Perhaps add some sweet potatoes to your omelet, or try our Raspberry and Apple Power Oatmeal on page 90. If exercising frequently for long durations, you may also need to increase your overall carbohydrate intake, as well as the number of servings across the day.

HOW MANY CARBOHYDRATES SHOULD YOU EAT?

The following illustrations provide a basic starting point for you to establish your optimal carbohydrate intake based on your body composition. **There are no rules set in stone, so these are just suggestions.**

Men

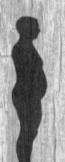

- ★ Maintain or build size
- ★ Consume carbohydrates frequently
- ★ 3-4 servings daily
- ★ **Sources:** Gluten free/pseudo grains, legumes, potatoes, fruit (whole, dried and juice) sweet potatoes and root vegetables

200-400G DAILY

- ★ Burn fat and build lean body mass
- ★ Moderate carbohydrate consumption
- ★ 1-3 servings daily
- ★ **Sources:** Gluten free/pseudo grains, legumes, potatoes, fruit (whole) sweet potatoes and root vegetables

150-250G DAILY

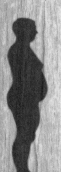

- ★ Lose large amount of body fat
- ★ Limit carbohydrate consumption
- ★ 1 serving after exercise or in the evening
- ★ **Sources:** berries, vegetables, legumes and root vegetables

50-100G DAILY

Women

★ Maintain weight and lean mass
★ Consume carbohydrates frequently
★ 3-4 servings daily
★ **Sources:** Gluten free/pseudo grains, legumes, potatoes, fruit (whole, dried and juice) sweet potatoes and root vegetables

200-300G DAILY

★ Lose little/maintain body fat, increase lean mass
★ Moderate carbohydrate consumption
★ 1-3 servings daily
★ **Sources:** Gluten free/pseudo grains, legumes, potatoes, fruit (whole) sweet potatoes and root vegetables

150-250G DAILY

★ Lose large amount of bodyfat
★ Limit carbohydrate consumption
★ 1 serving after exercise or in the evening
★ **Sources:** berries, legumes, vegetables and root vegetables

50-150G DAILY

Remember there are no rules set in stone, so these are just suggestions.

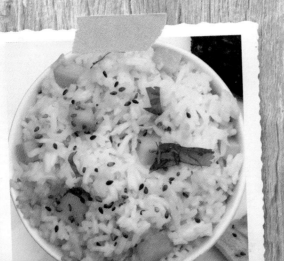

QUICK CARBOHYDRATE REFERENCE GUIDE

To keep this macro business simple again, here is a quick reference guide to help you manage your carbohydrate intake:

GRAINS, LEGUMES & PSEUDO GRAINS *Approximate values*

★ Rice, cooked (125g)	28g	★ 20 cashew nuts (28g)	9g
★ Quinoa, cooked (125g)	26g	★ 25 peanuts (28g)	4.6g
★ Peas, cooked (100g)	10.5g		

VEGETABLES

FYI, A POTATO NOT A POO!

★ 1 large white potato , baked (180g)	37g	★ Butternut squash, cooked (200g)	22g
★ 1 large sweet potato, baked (180g)	37g	★ 2 carrots, raw (120g)	12g
★ 6 new potatoes, boiled (200g)	32g	★ 1 medium zucchini (196g)	6g
★ 1 small sweet potato, baked (150g)	31g	★ 2 small beets, cooked (100g)	7g
★ 1 medium parsnip, cooked (150g)	26g		

FRUIT

★ 1 medium plantain, boiled (230g)	74g	★ 1 whole avocado (200g)	17g
★ 3 medjool dates	54g	★ 6 dried apricots	13g
★ 1 medium banana (118g)	27g	★ ¼ of cantaloupe melon (276g)	11.5g
★ 1 medium pear (178g)	27g	★ Strawberries (150g punnet)	9g
★ 1 medium apple (180g)	25g	★ Raspberries (150g punnet)	7g
★ Blueberries (150g punnet)	22g		

FAT INTAKE

Fats also provide a source of energy to the human body and aid the transportation of fat-soluble vitamins A, D, E and K around the body. Fats are highly satiating and can have a profound effect on regulating appetite and balancing blood sugar levels. Hopefully, after reading our first book and the myths in Chapter 2 you now confidently understand that saturated, monounsaturated and omega fatty acids can all make a healthy contribution to your nutritional intake.

An easy way to establish your fat intake is to work out your protein and carbohydrate needs first, and then source the remaining calories from... fat. See **Putting It All Together** on page 61 to understand how to do this.

BIG FAT TIP

We **LOVE** fats and they have some wonderful benefits, but as with any foods there is still a need for portion control. When using fats for cooking or dressing, to avoid tipping into calorie excess, add carefully with a spoon rather than just pouring huge amounts onto your food. The same goes for nuts and coconut milk. These are wonderful healthy fats but still require portion control.

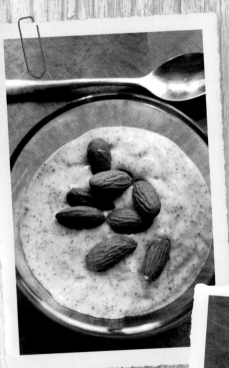

BALANCING FAT INTAKE

The following diagram is a quick reminder of how to balance your healthy fat intake.

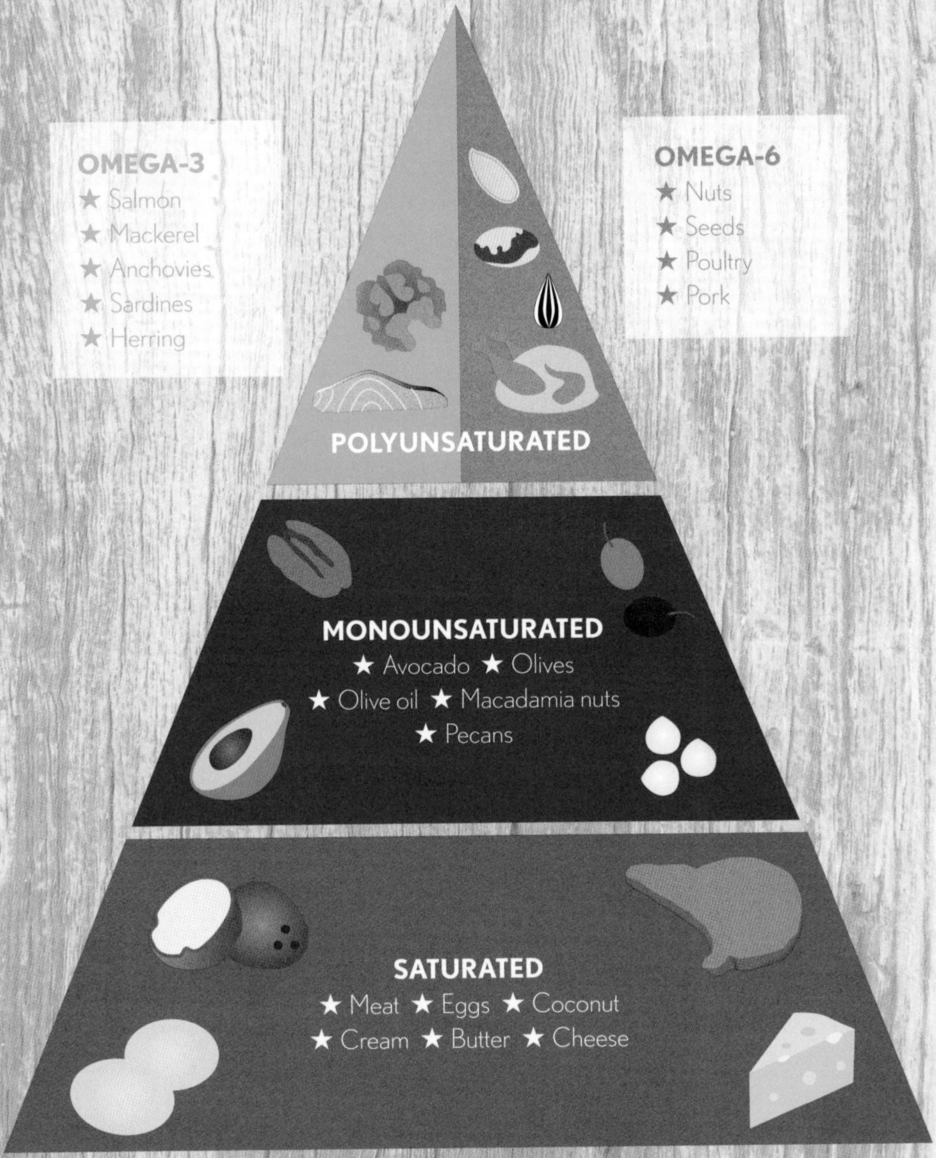

OMEGA-3
★ Salmon
★ Mackerel
★ Anchovies
★ Sardines
★ Herring

OMEGA-6
★ Nuts
★ Seeds
★ Poultry
★ Pork

POLYUNSATURATED

MONOUNSATURATED
★ Avocado ★ Olives
★ Olive oil ★ Macadamia nuts
★ Pecans

SATURATED
★ Meat ★ Eggs ★ Coconut
★ Cream ★ Butter ★ Cheese

QUICK FAT REFERENCE GUIDE

Here is a quick reference guide to help you manage your fat intake:

FAT SOURCE	PORTION SIZE *Approximate weight*	FAT CONTENT *Approximate values*
★ Almonds	20 nuts / 28g	14g
★ Almond butter	2 tablespoons / 32g	17.7g
★ Bacon	2 slices grilled / 38g	5.3g
★ Brazil nuts	6 nuts	19g
★ Beef	Ground (20% fat) / 100g	19.8g
★ Butter	2 tablespoons / 28g	22g
★ Cashews	20 nuts / 28g	12g
★ Cashew butter	2 tablespoons / 32g	15.9g
★ Coconut (desiccated)	2 tablespoons / 28g	18g
★ Coconut oil	1 tablespoon / 14g	14g
★ Chicken breast	1 fillet / 120g	4g
★ Chicken drumstick	2 drumsticks / 200g	18g
★ Chicken thigh	2-3 thighs / 100g	8-9g
★ Cottage cheese	3 tablespoons / 60g	4g
★ Double cream	2 tablespoons / 30g	15.2g
★ Eggs	1 medium	5g
★ Feta cheese	1 tablespoon / 28g	5g
★ Ham	1 slice / 24g	0.6g
★ Hazelnuts	20 nuts / 28g	17g
★ Lamb chop	2 chops, fat trimmed / 55g	15g
★ Lamb	Ground (20% fat) / 100g	19.8g
★ Lamb's liver	100g	6.2g
★ Macadamias	10-12 nuts / 28g	21g
★ Pork chop	1 chop, fat trimmed / 85g	10.3g
★ Tuna in olive oil	1 can / 160g	11g
★ Salmon	1 fillet / 130g	15.6g
★ Salmon	1 can / 213g	8g
★ Sardines	1 can in water / 120g	8g
★ Sardines	1 can in olive oil (drained) / 120g	12.6g
★ Pork sausage	2 sausages / (97% pork grilled) / 105g	28g
★ Sea bass	1 fillet / 72g	2.5g
★ Sirloin steak fillet	Fillet, fat trimmed / 135g	4g
★ Rump steak fillet	Fillet, fat trimmed / 160g	15.7g
★ Ribeye steak fillet	Fillet, fat trimmed / 121g	10.5g
★ Turkey	Ground thighs / 100g	5.6g
★ Yogurt (natural full-fat)	100g	4g
★ Walnuts	14 halves / 28g	18g

PUTTING IT ALL TOGETHER: A STEP-BY-STEP GUIDE

CALCULATE YOUR BMR

www.bmi-calculator.net/bmr-calculator/

↓

CALCULATE YOUR TOTAL CALORIE NEED INCLUDING PHYSICAL ACTIVITY

★ Little/no exercise: multiply BMR by **1.2**
★ Light exercise: multiply BMR by **1.375**
★ Moderate exercise: multiply BMR by **1.55**
★ Very active: multiply BMR by **1.725**
★ Extra active: multiply BMR by **1.9**

↓

CALCULATE YOUR MINIMUM PROTEIN REQUIREMENTS IN GRAMS AND MULTIPLY BY 4 TO CONVERT TO CALORIES

Sedentary/little exercise = **.54g** per pound of bodyweight
Regular endurance/gym based exercise = **.68g** per pound of bodyweight
Strength/hypertrophy training = **.82g** per pound of bodyweight

↓

DECIDE ON A CARBOHYDRATE INTAKE BASED UPON THE GUIDANCE IN THIS CHAPTER.

We suggest most people start around .9g/lb and experiment from there. Multiply the number by 4 to convert to calories

↓

FATS CAN NOW MAKE UP THE REMAINING CALORIES:

Total calorie target -> minus protein calories -> minus carbohydrate calories = fat calories
To convert back into grams divide by 9.

Revisit the calorie flowchart on page 49 if you wish to monitor your progress.

EASY PEASY MACROS AND PORTIONS

If you're feeling overwhelmed with all the information on macronutrients, then simply take our favorite Fitter Food approach, and keep it simple. You can use your hand as a guide for portion control:

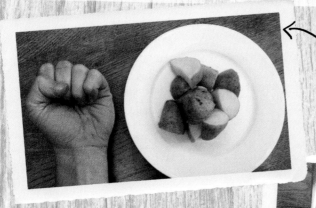

★ A fist-sized serving of starch-based carbohydrates, e.g. potatoes, sweet potatoes, rice or quinoa

★ Plus two handfuls of non-starchy vegetables, e.g. spinach, peppers, zucchini or salad leaves

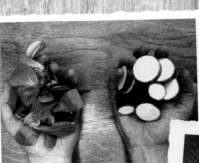

★ Spoonful of added fat, e.g. olive oil, cheese or nuts

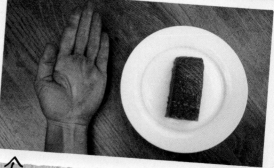

TIP

Men looking to build lean body mass and participating in exercise may wish to double these portion sizes or add an extra meal to daily intake.

★ A palm-sized serving of protein, e.g. fillet of fish, chicken breast or steak

MEAL TIMING & SNACKS

When you make any significant changes to your nutrition, it's important to keep your blood sugar levels stable to avoid energy crashes, cravings and feeling too hungry. Each of these has the potential to derail your healthy intentions. The following tips provide a good basis to start with, which you can then adapt based upon the results:

1 Start by having a breakfast, lunch and dinner.

2 We advise most people to reduce snacking and actually increase the gaps between meals to encourage the body to burn fat for fuel and rest the digestive system. Don't get too carried away with this; once blood sugar levels are balanced most people benefit from having 4-5 hours between meals.

3 Given the long working days most of us endure, many people have lunch at midday and don't eat again until late in the evening. In this case at least one snack or extra small meal may be necessary especially around 3:30-4:30 pm when the body's energy levels naturally begin to dip.

4 On the days you participate in exercise or are generally more active, add 1-2 extra small meals or snacks. You may require more carbohydrates on these days.

5 Fast for 12 hours overnight to support immune health and hormone function. This may mean having an earlier evening meal or a slightly later breakfast.

6 Try to allow a 2-3 hour gap between your last meal and sleeping to optimize sleep health. You should be sleeping, not digesting.

SNACK IDEAS

- ★ Half an avocado
- ★ Piece of fruit
- ★ 12 raw nuts
- ★ Vegetable sticks and nut butter
- ★ Boiled eggs
- ★ Canned fish
- ★ Homemade burger or fishcake
- ★ Homemade soup or broth
- ★ Coconut chips

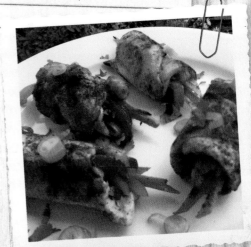

SEE OUR SNACK SUGGESTIONS ON PAGES 214-231.

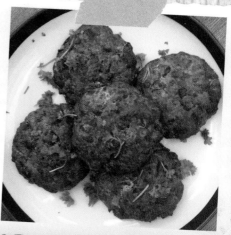

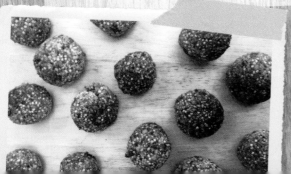

CHAPTER 6

Fitter Food's Ten Healthy Habits Of Success

When it comes to achieving long-term success with your goals, the key is integrating the information into your daily habits. When smarter choices become more habitual, you can high five yourself, because now you're **living** a healthy lifestyle. You have established what works for you and enjoy implementing it. Over the years you might make mistakes, but what's important is that you learn from the process.

The following are the healthy habits we firmly believe will have an incredibly positive effect on your health, mindset, body composition, energy levels, training and recovery. We don't expect you to put them all in place straight away; just take small steps in your own time.

1. Eat single-ingredient, home-cooked food 80% of the time.

This quite simply means eating food that has not undergone any form of processing; food in its purest form. If it has a label, you could already be in the wrong supermarket aisle. If you don't recognize the ingredients, you are definitely in the wrong supermarket aisle! As well as sourcing your own ingredients, you also need to cook them yourself, otherwise you miss out on the **cephalic** phase of digestion. Basically, when you prepare food and release its wonderful aromas, your senses detect that good stuff is coming and kick the digestive system into action. This releases enzymes and stomach acid; a vital step to ensure you break down and absorb nutrients.

It is also vital you do not rush the eating process. You must relax, chew your food properly and taste each bite. Use a knife as well as a fork, rather than shovelling food in with a **FORKLIFT**. Slowing down your body in this way at mealtimes also puts it into **'REST AND DIGEST'** mode whereby all the digestive hormones are switched on and it is ready to break down your food.

WHAT DOES 80% LOOK LIKE?

In terms of establishing what 80% looks like, count how many meals and snacks you have across a week:

Daily = 3 meals, 1 snack ➜ Weekly = 28 meals/snacks
80% = 0.8 x 28 = 22.4

Therefore 23 (round it up) of your meals/snacks need to be highly nutritious and 5 meals/snacks can be more flexible.

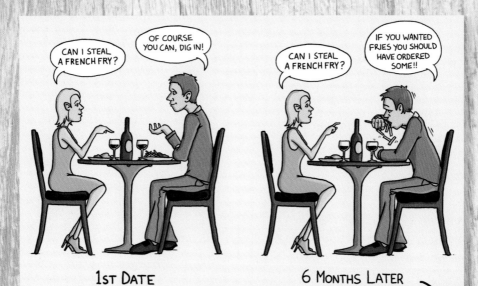

1ST DATE

6 MONTHS LATER

If you are addressing some health issues and need to focus a little more on nutrient density and elimination, you may wish to adopt a 90% approach:

$$90\% = 0.9 \times 28 = 25$$

25 of your meals/snacks need to highly nutritious and 3 meals or snacks can be more flexible.

EAT LIKE YOU'RE ON A FIRST DATE, POLITELY AND SLOWLY, CHEWING FOOD AND USING A KNIFE AND FORK.

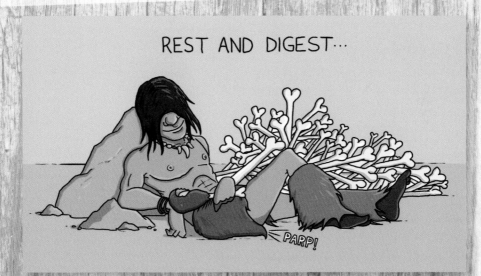

REST AND DIGEST...

"Habit is habit, and not to be flung out of the window by any man, but coaxed down-stairs one step at a time." **MARK TWAIN**

2. Get 7–9 hours' sleep each night.

The more good-quality sleep, you get the better you feel. It's not always possible but try your best, as sleep is the **"MacDaddy of health and fat loss."** While you sleep, your body has the opportunity to assess the damage of the day and do what is required to restore balance. Ideally you should always wake up with renewed energy and positivity, ready to face the day.

Sleep health is also a vital part of your fat loss goals, as sleep deprivation decreases insulin sensitivity. Lack of sleep also increases ghrelin, the hormone responsible for appetite. Have you ever noticed how ravenous you feel after a terrible night's sleep?

QUICK TIPS FOR A BETTER NIGHT'S SLEEP

✔ Limit caffeine consumption or completely eliminate it if you have any sleep issues.

✔ Switch off phones, computers and bright lights after sunset, and ideally by 9 pm. This will support the release of the sleep hormone, melatonin.

✔ Unwind by watching some comedy, a film or use some of the stress management activities detailed below.

✔ Don't eat too late. You should be sleeping, not digesting.

✔ Have an Epsom salts bath. This provides a dose of the calming mineral magnesium. Combine with some lavender candles and you'll be sleeping like a baby.

✔ Establish a routine where you go to bed and get up at a similar time each day, even on the weekends. This allows your waking and sleeping hormones to get into a natural rhythm. Eventually you might not even need an alarm.

✔ Get a bit frisky, and if they pull the "too tired" card, tell them it will enhance the quality of their sleep. **BOSH!**

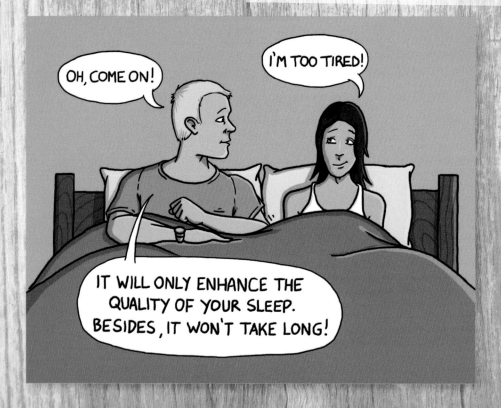

3. Listen to your body to discover what works for you.

This is a really important habit to master, and something many people miss. What works for one person may not work for another, and with so much information out there it's easy to get confused. There are so many variables to take into account, including age, sex, race, genes and lifestyle factors. However, your biggest ally here is your own body. It's clever, and great at telling you when it's happy and when it's not. We covered **Signs Your Diet Isn't Working** in our first book, discussing the importance of assessing feedback like bloating, fatigue, bad skin or a consistent lack of results. Equally, when something is working for you, don't be distracted or tempted from your path just because you've read or heard about an alternative approach. Stick to your own success.

4. Perform ten minutes of active stress management a day.

Our bodies are designed to cope with short, sharp bursts of stress by switching into **"fight or flight mode,"** which is fuelled by our stress hormones cortisol and adrenaline.

Historically, this would have been our survival mode when faced with a life threatening experience. However, a ticking time bomb for many of us is the way we spend our entire day in "fight or flight mode." Unlike our ancestors, we're not challenged by famine or running from wild animals. Instead, our stress triggers are travel delays, road rage, computers saying 'no' and ill-mannered people we encounter throughout our day. In some ways they present a greater threat with their chronic, persistent nature.

While you cannot remove many of these things from your life, you can buffer the impact they have on your health with some active stress management each day. All of the following have been shown to lower the production of stress hormones and ease the body out of "fight or flight" mode.

ACTIVE STRESS MANAGEMENT

- ✔ A ten-minute walk outdoors
- ✔ Listening to relaxing music or a podcast
- ✔ Reading a book
- ✔ Calling an understanding friend
- ✔ A ten-minute power nap
- ✔ Ten minutes of slow, deep breathing
- ✔ Mindful activities like puzzles, coloring, drawing or other craft-based hobbies
- ✔ Meditation

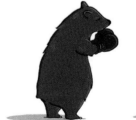

FIGHT....
OR FLIGHT ?

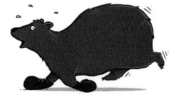

5. Limit caffeine.

The main sources of caffeine on the Fitter Food pyramid are tea, coffee and dark chocolate. While the health benefits of these mean they can make a positive contribution to your nutrition, it's important to remain in control of stimulant consumption. If you cannot physically start your day without a caffeine hit, this needs to be addressed, and it's advisable to remove it for a short period of time to optimize your energy levels before reintroducing it. Similarly, if you have sleep issues, consider eliminating caffeine to assess the impact it may be having. If you enjoy these foods and don't wish to miss out on the antioxidant content and prebiotic effect they have on our gut bacteria, they can be reintroduced once you are no longer 'dependent' on them. In the meantime you can drink naturally decaffeinated varieties (usually labelled Swiss water or CO_2-processed). With tea, coffee and chocolate, choosing organic will likely offer greater benefits, as extensive amounts of pesticides and fertilizers are used in cultivating these foods.

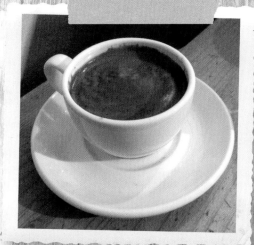

6. Limit alcohol.

We're not suggesting you live like a monk; we live in the real world and always encourage balance. A little wine or a couple of beers here and there is fine if your body tolerates the ingredients. Studies have shown that drinking in moderation may be healthier than abstaining completely from alcohol, but these observations may also be due to the fact that people who drink in moderation generally lead a healthier lifestyle— moderation is not a word in everyone's vocabulary. Only you know where you sit with this.

We only tend to drink alcohol on social occasions, and stick to 1-2 servings. Any more than this won't do your waistline or wallet any favors. Alcohol disrupts insulin health, and the detoxification process depletes essential vitamins and minerals. Plus most alcoholic beverages pack in a lot of calories and sugar. And beers and ales also contain gluten. Quality can be significant too, and therefore biodynamic wine, craft beers and traditionally-distilled spirits may be lower in additives and a little easier on the system.

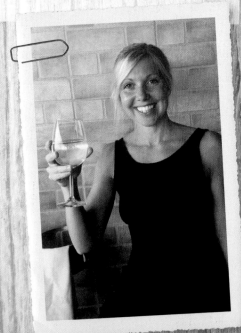

7. Exercise 2-5 times a week.

The key with exercise is to find something you enjoy. This ensures that you will be consistent in your routine and continue to make progress. The fitness industry is often harping on about a new bit of equipment or training method, telling people what they should and should not be doing, all the while just generally confusing people. The key is that your heart rate gets elevated a couple of times a week and you work your muscles.

Never take movement for granted. Discover your body's abilities and make the most of them. You can squat, push, pull, run, sprint and jump. Step out of your comfort zone from time-to-time—it's character-building and incredibly rewarding. We often suggest that people take up a skill-based exercise so it's no longer just a workout; instead it involves learning and striving for better performance. Some great examples include boxing, rock climbing, gymnastics, Olympic lifting, power lifting, tennis, badminton or any kind of team sport.

It's important to note that there is a dose-response curve with exercise as illustrated below. Just enough supports good health, but in excess immune function is suppressed, essential nutrients are depleted and hormonal balance may be disrupted. We suggest experimenting with 2-5 exercise sessions a week (around 45-60 minutes in duration). And remember—the more you exercise, the more recovery you need.

Hard Work + Enjoyment + Consistency = Progression and Results

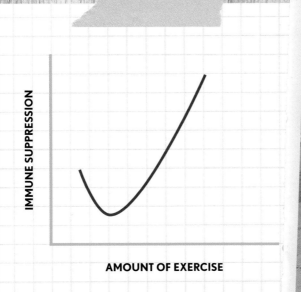

IMMUNE SUPPRESSION

AMOUNT OF EXERCISE

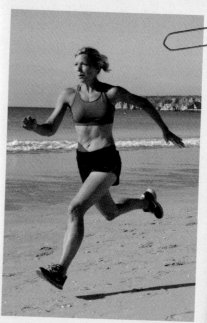

8. Move daily.

There is a difference between movement and exercise. The human body is designed to change positions and move lightly throughout the day by walking, standing, squatting and moving across different terrains such as stairs—remember those?

The irony is that incorporating movement into your day is much easier than going to the gym. No sports kit required; no shower or warm up, you just **MOVE**. Yet many of us fail to do this on a regular basis.

Movement energizes you, aids recovery from exercise, improves sleep health and increases **NEAT** which stands for **Non-Exercise Activity Thermogenesis**. This is the energy you burn when not sleeping, eating or exercising. Sitting is the new smoking, so get on up off that chair and do something.

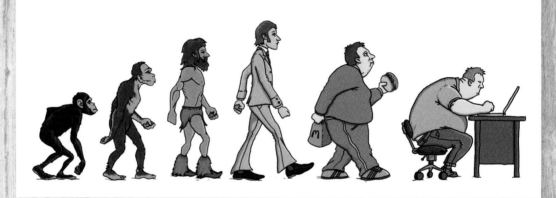

TIPS ON MOVING MORE

✔ Actually go shopping rather than clicking items online and sitting on the sofa waiting for a delivery.
✔ Use a shopping basket instead of a cart.
✔ Walk part of your commute or take a stroll on your lunch hour.
✔ Ditch labor-saving devices and services to do your own cleaning, gardening and DIY jobs.
✔ Do some bodyweight squats or push-ups every time you go to the bathroom.
✔ Check out the 100 Rep Challenge for some inspiration on how to incorporate more movement into your day: www.100repchallenge.com
✔ Do a four-minute dance tabata: 20 seconds of energetic dance moves to your favorite tunes, followed by 10 seconds resting for 8 rounds.

#dancetabata

WARNING THIS IS FUN!!

9. Treat yourself occasionally.

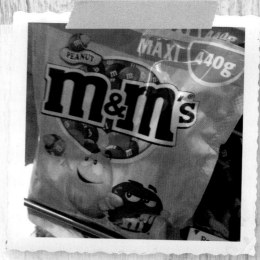

You will notice the top of the Fitter Food pyramid includes **"a little of what you fancy."** Yes, that's right; we're suggesting you treat yourself occasionally. It might be a pizza, ice cream or your favorite chocolate bar or cake. We're not suggesting these should be paleo-ish, guilt-free, low fat or gluten-free either, unless of course you can't tolerate certain ingredients.

The key is ensuring they remain on the **occasional list** so that what you consume 80% of the time has the biggest impact on your health and fat loss goals. Allowing yourself this freedom removes any sense of restriction, and you will be able to develop a new appreciation for these foods. Most importantly, finding this balance ensures you maintain a healthy relationship with food.

10. Fast for 12 hours overnight.

The research on fasting is still in its infancy, not to mention the number of variables that need to be accounted for. Nutrition status varies significantly across individuals, and while one person might get epic results from fasting, another might experience weight gain and fatigue. Your daily routine and relationship with food are also relevant. If you're working excessively long hours, participating in frequent intense exercise or have a history of disordered eating, fasting may have a negative impact upon your health.

There are some studies indicating that going for extended periods of time without food can support fat loss, disease prevention and longevity. One of the easiest ways you can benefit from this with little intrusion to your lifestyle is to extend your overnight fast. That way you sleep through most of the experience. It really just involves having an earlier dinner or slightly later breakfast. For instance, if you eat dinner at 8 pm then don't eat breakfast until 8 am.

Feel free to experiment with other models of fasting. We generally find that having a 12-hour fast overnight, or skipping the odd meal if we're busy, keeps this fasting business easy and uncomplicated.

Aim to incorporate these habits into your day as much as you can. Find a way to make them work for you and your schedule. By simply getting more sleep, moving more and reducing processed food consumption, you will make a HUGE difference in your body composition, health and happiness.

CHAPTER 7
Tools To Get You Started

PANTRY

Here are some cupboard essentials that are handy to have in stock as many of these ingredients are used in Fitter Food recipes.

FATS
Oils
- [ ] Avocado oil
- [ ] Extra virgin coconut oil
- [ ] Extra virgin olive oil
- [ ] Macadamia oil

Solid Fats
- [ ] Ghee
- [ ] Grass-fed butter
- [ ] Coconut cream (can or carton)
- [ ] Coconut manna
- [ ] Creamed coconut (bar)

Nuts/Nut Butters/Nut Milks
- [ ] Almond
- [ ] Brazil
- [ ] Cashews
- [ ] Chestnuts
- [ ] Coconut
- [ ] Hazelnuts
- [ ] Macadamias
- [ ] Pecans
- [ ] Pistachios
- [ ] Walnuts

Seeds/Seed Butters
- [ ] Chia
- [ ] Flaxseed
- [ ] Hemp
- [ ] Pumpkin

PROTEINS
Poultry/Eggs (ideally free range, grass-fed or organic)
- [ ] Chicken
- [ ] Duck
- [ ] Goose
- [ ] Turkey

Meat/Game (ideally free range, grass-fed or organic)
- [ ] Beef
- [ ] Buffalo
- [ ] Game
- [ ] Gluten-free sausages (more than 80% meat)
- [ ] Lamb
- [ ] Organ meats (liver and kidney)
- [ ] Pheasant
- [ ] Pork
- [ ] Venison

Fish/Seafood
- [ ] Anchovies
- [ ] Bream
- [ ] Cod
- [ ] Coley
- [ ] Haddock
- [ ] Herring
- [ ] Mackerel
- [ ] Pollock
- [ ] Salmon
- [ ] Sardines
- [ ] Scallops
- [ ] Sea bass
- [ ] Shrimp
- [ ] Squid
- [ ] Trout

CARBOHYDRATES
Starches
- [ ] White potatoes
- [ ] Sweet potatoes
- [ ] Root vegetables (celery root, turnips, rutabaga, parsnips)
- [ ] Plantains
- [ ] Cassava/Tapioca
- [ ] White or wild rice
- [ ] Quinoa

Vegetables
- [ ] Artichoke
- [ ] Arugula
- [ ] Asparagus
- [ ] Broccoli
- [ ] Brussels sprouts
- [ ] Butternut squash
- [ ] Cabbage
- [ ] Carrots
- [ ] Cauliflower
- [ ] Celery
- [ ] Celery root
- [ ] Cucumber
- [ ] Eggplant
- [ ] Kale
- [ ] Leeks
- [ ] Lettuce
- [ ] Mushrooms
- [ ] Parsnips
- [ ] Peppers
- [ ] Radish
- [ ] Red onions
- [ ] Spinach
- [ ] Swiss chard
- [ ] Watercress
- [ ] White onions
- [ ] Zucchini

Fruit
Favor low-sugar fruits:
- [ ] Lemons/Limes
- [ ] Avocados
- [ ] Berries
- [ ] Tomatoes (sauce and purée)

Rotate all other fruits
Have 1–3 servings daily

OTHER
Herbs and spices
- [ ] All

Miscellaneous
- [ ] Coconut flour
- [ ] Rice flour
- [ ] Tapioca flour
- [ ] Xylitol
- [ ] Raw honey
- [ ] Stevia
- [ ] Coconut palm sugar
- [ ] Cocoa
- [ ] Vanilla extract
- [ ] Apple cider vinegar
- [ ] Organic cane sugar

DRINKS
- [ ] Coconut water (no added sugar)
- [ ] Mineral/filtered water
- [ ] Green, black or white leaf tea
- [ ] Herbal teas
- [ ] Unsweetened nut milks

PROTEIN POWDERS

We often use protein supplements for pure convenience. A protein smoothie is a great meal or snack if you are short on time. We encourage you to source a good quality protein powder with minimal ingredients, preferably one that uses natural sweeteners. Below we've listed some trusted brands:

FLAVORED POWDERS
- [ ] Dr Mercola (Whey)
- [ ] Jarrow Formulas (Rice or Whey)
- [ ] Nutri Advanced UltraPro Whey (Whey)
- [ ] Rawlicious (Rice, Hemp, Pea)
- [ ] Solgar Whey To Go (Whey)
- [ ] Sunwarrior (Rice)
- [ ] Vega One (Rice, Hemp, Pea)
- [ ] Vega Sport (Rice, Hemp, Pea)
- [ ] Vital Protein (pea protein)

UNFLAVORED POWDERS
- [ ] Good Hemp Protein
- [ ] Dr Mercola 100% Pure Pea Protein
- [ ] Now Foods Whey
- [ ] Pulsin Whey, Rice, Hemp or Pea
- [ ] The Organic Protein Company

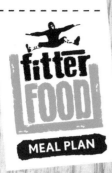

FITTER FOOD

MEAL PLAN

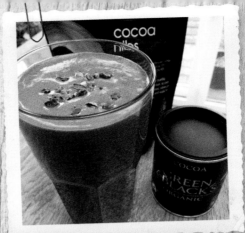

DAY 1

BREAKFAST
Cottage Flaxcakes
(page 97)

LUNCH
Tomato and Tarragon
Soup with Epic
Herby Salad
(pages 116 and 203)

DINNER
Greek Salad Burgers
with Quick Carrot and
Cilantro Slaw and rice
(pages 158 and 195)

DAY 2

BREAKFAST
Turkey Toast Toppers
(page 99)

LUNCH
Leftover Greek Salad
Burgers with salad

DINNER
Curried Fish Bake with
potatoes and steamed
vegetables
(page 135)

DAY 3

BREAKFAST
Mint Choc Chip
smoothie
(page 104)

LUNCH
Leftover Tomato
and Tarragon Soup

DINNER
Smoky Pork Meatballs
with zucchini
(page 153)

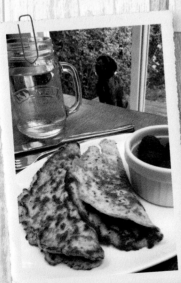

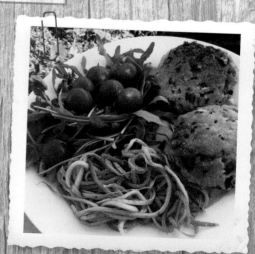

DAY 4

BREAKFAST
Avocado and
Salmon Calzone
(page 83)

LUNCH
Leftover Smoky Pork
Meatballs with salad

DINNER
Smoky Salmon Burgers
with steamed sweet
potatoes, mixed
salad and homemade
guacamole
(page 164)

DAY 5

BREAKFAST
Green Machine
smoothie
(page 106)

LUNCH
Leftover Salmon
Burgers with salad

DINNER
Paella Pronto with salad
(page 133)

DAY 6

BREAKFAST
Protein Pancakes
(page 84)

LUNCH
Goji Greens Salad
(page 201)

DINNER
Mini Protein Pizzas with
Crinkle Cut Sesame Sweet
Pot Chips and salad
(pages 144 and 194)

DAY 7

BREAKFAST
Eggs in Avo Boats
(page 92)

LUNCH
Leftover Protein Pizzas
with salad

DINNER
Balsamic Roast Chicken
with Super Mash and
steamed vegetables
(pages 178 and 191)

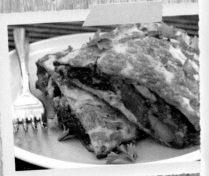

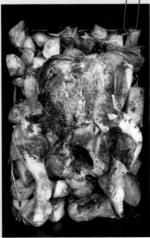

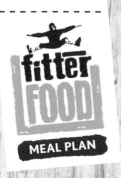

fitter FOOD

MEAL PLAN

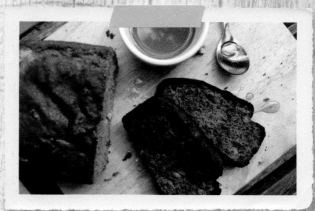

DAY 8

BREAKFAST
Fitter Breakfast Wrap filled with smoked salmon, spinach and egg (page 93)

LUNCH
Leftover Balsamic Roast Chicken with salad

DINNER
Beef 5 A Day Stir Fry with white rice (page 148)

DAY 9

BREAKFAST
Hidden Greens smoothie (page 105)

LUNCH
Leftover Beef 5 A Day Stir Fry

DINNER
Marinated Garlic, Honey and Mustard Salmon with new potatoes and steamed spinach (page 125)

DAY 10

BREAKFAST
Salty Banana Cinnamon Scramble (page 98)

LUNCH
Leftover Honey and Mustard Salmon and salad

DINNER
Spanish Style Chicken with steamed broccoli and green beans (page 142)

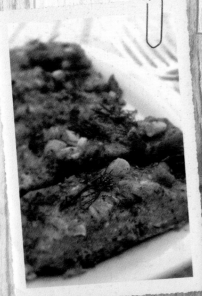

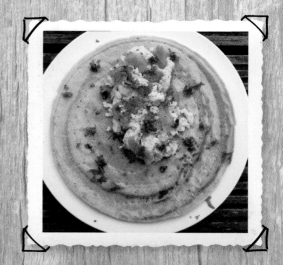

Aim to have a big salad each day and a couple of portions of non-starchy vegetables with each meal

DAY 11

BREAKFAST
Raspberry and Apple Power Oatmeal
(page 90)

LUNCH
Leftover Spanish Style Chicken

DINNER
Fish in a Thai Bag with a baked sweet potato and steamed kale
(page 122)

DAY 12

BREAKFAST
Banana Bread smoothie
(page 106)

LUNCH
Pimp a salad
(page 198)

DINNER
Seafood Tandoori Mixed Grill with rice and salad
(page 126)

DAY 13

BREAKFAST
Brunch Loaf
(page 87)

LUNCH
Hulk Soup
(page 111)

DINNER
Fish, Chips and Mushy Pea Cakes with roasted vegetables and Tartar Sauce
(pages 132 and 227)

DAY 14

BREAKFAST
Sweet Potato Hash Browns with fried eggs and spinach
(page 89)

LUNCH
Hulk Soup

DINNER
Butternut Squash Lasagna with salad
(page 180)

RESOURCES

AWESOME WEBSITES IN THE USA
Exercise and Nutrition

★ 100 Rep Challenge: Excellence Is A Habit
www.100repchallenge.com

★ Charles Poliquin Official Website
www.strengthsensei.com

★ Chris Kresser: Let's Take Back Your Health
www.chriskresser.com
www.kresserinstitute.com

★ Dr Ragnar – Health and Fitness In The
Real World (Aka Tommy Wood)
www.drragnar.com

★ Marks Daily Apple
www.marksdailyapple.com

★ Robb Wolf: Revolutionary Solutions
To Modern Life
www.robbwolf.com

★ Soberistas: Love Life In Control
www.soberistas.com

GREAT PLACES TO SHOP

★ Premier Organics - Nuts and nut butters
www.premierorganics.org

★ Au Bon Broth - Bone broth
www.aubonbroth.com

★ Bare Bones - Bone broth
www.barebonesbroth.com

★ Santa Barbara Chocolate
www.santabarbarachocolate.com

★ Caveman Coffee - Coffee and tea
www.cavemancoffeeco.com

★ Eating Evolved
www.eatingevolved.com

★ Paleo Treats
www.paleotreats.com

★ Nikki's Coconut Butter
www.nikkiscoconutbutter.com

★ Wise Choice Market
www.wisechoicemarket.com

★ Tropical Traditions - Coconut oil
www.tropicaltraditions.com

★ Pure Indian Foods - Ghee
www.pureindianfoods.com

★ Lucero - Olive oil
www.luceerooliveoil.com

SOURCING INGREDIENTS
Sourcing local ingredients will ensure your
nutrition has a higher nutrient content. If there
is nothing convenient to you locally, then
consider buying directly from a farm online
or use online food delivery companies. The
following are helpful resources and suppliers.

MEAT SUPPLIERS

★ Diestal Turkey Ranch
www.diestelturkey.com

★ Brandon Natural Beef
www.brandonnaturalbeef.com

★ Nick's Sticks - Beef and turkey sticks
www.nicks-sticks.com

★ Get Maine Lobster
www.getmainelobster.com

★ Primal Pastures
www.primalpastures.com

★ Safe Catch - Lowest mercury canned tuna
www.safecatch.com

★ Tendergrass Farms - Organic bacon
www.tendergrass.com

★ Thompson River Ranch
www.thompsonriverranch.com

★ TX Organics
www.txbarorganics.com

★ Wild Pacific Salmon
www.wildpacificsalmon.com

FARMER'S MARKETS

★ Local Harvest - Find a farmer's market near you
www.localharvest.org

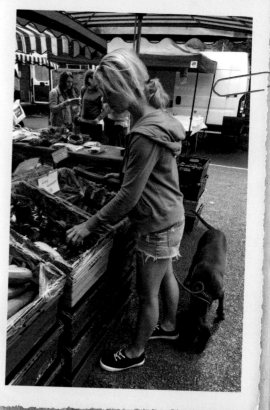

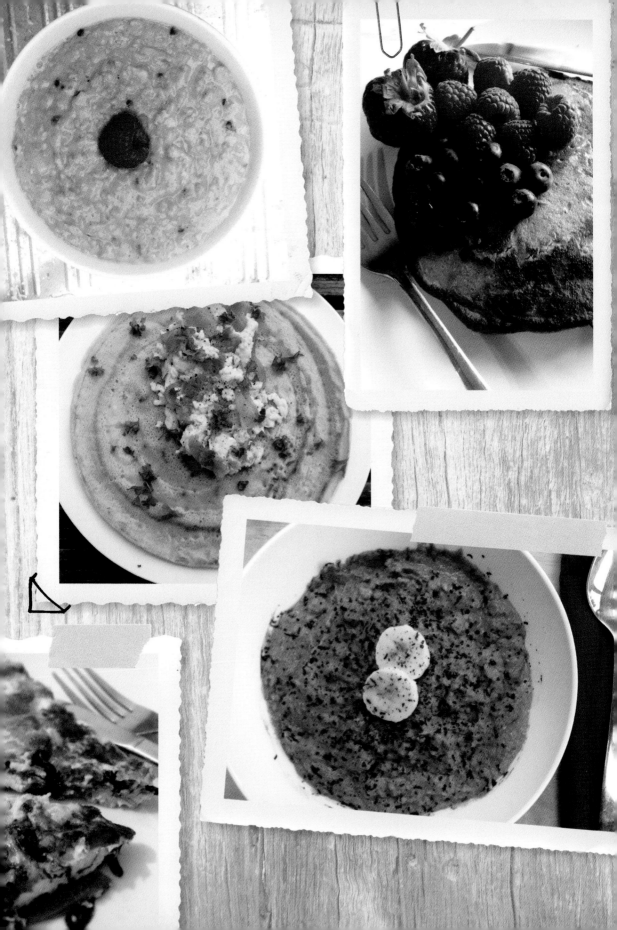

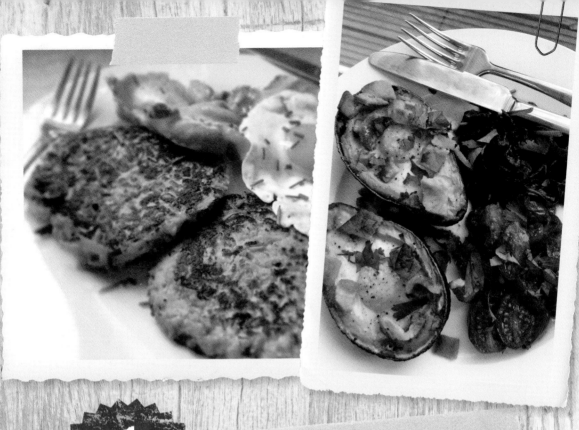

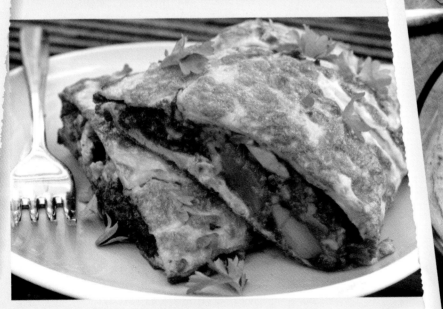

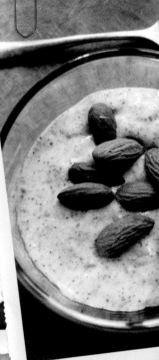

1 Breakfasts

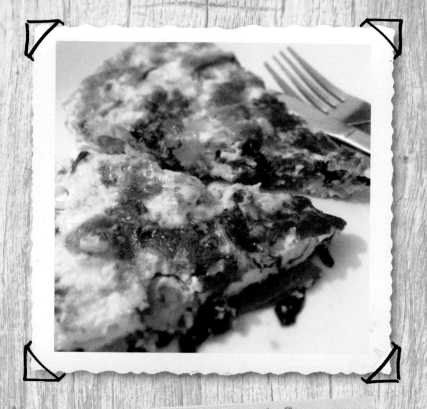

English Breakfast Frittata

Ingredients

★ 1 tbsp coconut oil , olive oil or butter for cooking
★ 4 gluten-free sausages, chopped
★ 4 slices bacon, chopped
★ 4 tomatoes, chopped
★ 1 handful spinach
★ 10 eggs, beaten

1 Heat the oil in a pan over a medium heat and then add the sausages and bacon. Cook for 3-4 minutes before adding the tomatoes.

2 Cook and stir occasionally for another 3-4 minutes or until the tomatoes have softened, then add the spinach and stir fry.

3 Once the spinach has wilted, add the eggs to the pan and push the ingredients around a bit to allow the egg to get right to the bottom of the pan.

4 Preheat the grill.

5 Cook the eggs for about 4-5 minutes until the bottom half is fully cooked.

6 Place the pan under the grill (be careful not to melt the handle!) and leave until the frittata is a little golden on top and fully cooked in the middle. Be sure to keep an eye on it.

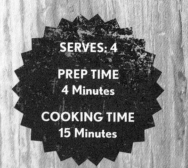

SERVES: 4

PREP TIME
4 Minutes

COOKING TIME
15 Minutes

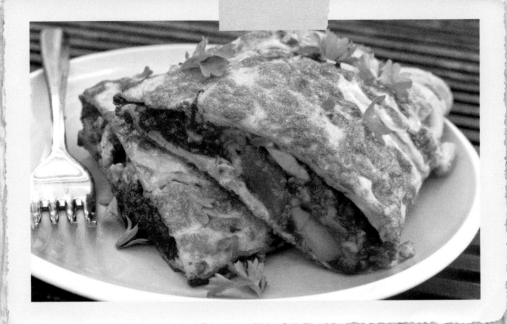

Avocado and Salmon Calzone

Ingredients
★ 4 eggs
★ ½ avocado, sliced
★ 2 oz (60g) smoked salmon, chopped
★ 1 large handful spinach
★ 2 heaped tbsp tomato purée
★ ½ tsp dried mixed herbs
★ Celtic Sea salt or Himalayan Pink salt and freshly ground black pepper
★ Coconut oil , olive oil or butter for cooking

SERVES: 2

PREP TIME
2 Minutes

COOKING TIME
8-10 Minutes

1 Melt a teaspoon of oil in a pan.

2 Beat the eggs in a large bowl until whites and yolks are mixed. Pour the mixture into the pan.

3 Leave to cook and use a spatula to gently peel away from the edges of the pan to ensure it doesn't stick.

4 Allow to cook through for a few minutes so the egg has set (it should be slightly runny on top).

5 Spread the tomato purée over the omelet base as if it was a pizza.

6 Tear up the spinach leaves and sprinkle these onto the cooked omelet. Add the avocado, salmon, herbs and seasoning and gently fold the omelet in half and seal the edges by pressing down with the spatula.

7 Allow to cook for another 5 minutes until the spinach has wilted.

8 This is best served hot from the pan, but like pizza is just as tasty served cold.

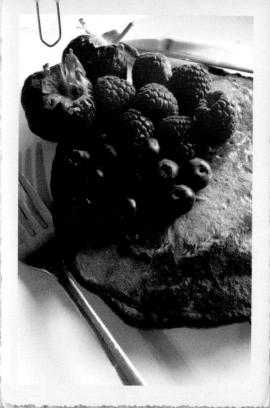

Protein Pancakes

Ingredients

★ 1 banana, mashed
★ 1 egg
★ 4 tsp (20g) vanilla protein powder
   (or substitute 2 more eggs)
★ 1 tbsp ground flaxseed
★ ¼ tsp vanilla extract
★ Coconut oil or butter for cooking

TO SERVE

★ Fresh berries and cinnamon
★ 1 tbsp cashew butter (optional)

1 Mix the ingredients thoroughly to make a batter (we used our Nutribullet blender).

2 Melt some coconut oil or butter in a non-stick frying pan.

3 Pour the batter into the pan and cook over medium-low heat for 2-3 minutes on one side until browned. Flip over and cook for another 3 minutes. You may wish to make 2-3 smaller pancakes as these will be easier to flip.

4 Top with fresh berries and cinnamon.

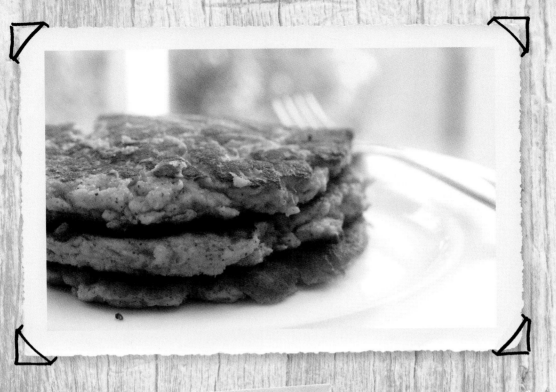

Sweet Pot Pancakes

Ingredients

★ 2 medium sweet potatoes, peeled, cooked and mashed (or use leftovers)
★ 3 eggs
★ 1 tsp vanilla extract
★ 2 heaped tbsp tapioca flour
★ 1 heaped tbsp coconut flour
★ ½ tsp baking powder
★ 1 tsp ground nutmeg
★ 1 tsp ground cinnamon
★ 2 tbsp coconut oil or butter for cooking

MAKES:
6-8 Pancakes

PREP TIME
15 Minutes

COOKING TIME
10 Minutes

1 Mix the sweet potato, eggs and vanilla extract.

2 In a separate bowl, use a fork to mix the tapioca flour, coconut flour, baking powder, nutmeg and cinnamon.

3 Gradually add the dry ingredients to the wet in small batches, stirring well each time, until a thick batter has formed.

4 Melt a little coconut oil or butter in a frying pan.

5 Place two tablespoons of batter in the pan and flatten slightly. Cook over a medium heat for 2-3 minutes and use a large spatula to flip the pancakes.

6 Press the top of the pancake with the spatula so you have the thickness and shape of a pancake. Cook for another 1-2 minutes on this side.

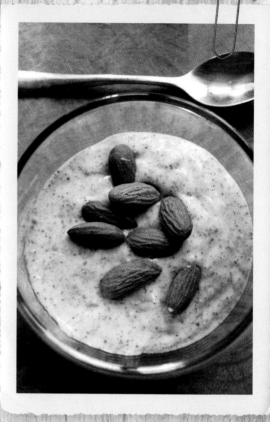

Chia Banana Porridge

Ingredients

★ 3 tbsp white or
  black chia seeds
★ ⅔ cup (150 ml) unsweetened
  coconut milk or almond milk
★ 1 tsp vanilla extract
★ A sprinkle of ground cinnamon
★ 2 tsp xylitol and raw honey
★ 1 ripe banana
★ 1 heaped tsp cashew butter

OPTIONAL EXTRAS

★ 1 tbsp raw nuts or seeds
★ 4 tbsp (20g) protein powder
★ 1 tbsp desiccated coconut

1 In a bowl, stir together the chia seeds, milk, vanilla, cinnamon and xylitol. Allow to sit for 15 minutes, or even better, refrigerate overnight.

2 The chia seeds will expand and absorb the liquid, creating a chia tapioca.

3 Mash a ripe banana in a bowl (or ideally use a blender) and combine thoroughly with the cashew butter.

4 NOTE: If you are not keen on tapioca texture, add the chia seeds to the blender to make the porridge a smoother consistency.

5 Melt a little coconut oil in a pan and add all the ingredients. Mix well and gently warm through.

6 Top with nuts, seeds, berries or coconut before serving, and stir in protein powder if desired.

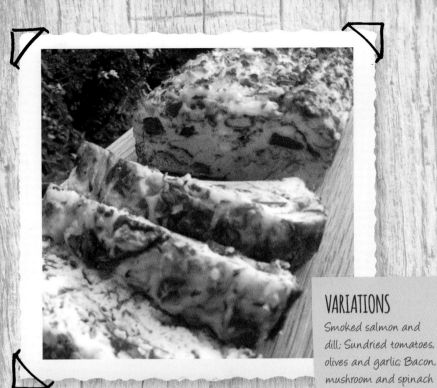

VARIATIONS

Smoked salmon and dill; Sundried tomatoes, olives and garlic; Bacon, mushroom and spinach

Brunch Loaf

Ingredients

★ 10 eggs
★ 1 zucchini
★ 1 handful spinach, chopped
★ 3.5 oz (100g) feta cheese, crumbled (optional)
★ 3 tbsp sundried tomatoes, drained and chopped
★ 2 tbsp fresh parsley, chopped

SERVES: 4-6

PREP TIME
10 Minutes

COOKING TIME
40-60 Minutes

1 Preheat the oven to 350°F.

2 Place the eggs in a large bowl and beat. For a lighter loaf, whisk the eggs with a mixer until pale and frothy.

3 Grate the zucchini directly into the beaten egg and fold in with a spoon.

5 Stir in the spinach, parsley, sundried tomatoes and most of the feta, but save a little to sprinkle on top of the loaf. Mix well.

6 This is optional, but if you prefer a lighter loaf add in a teaspoon of baking soda.

7 Line a loaf pan with parchment paper or grease with butter/coconut oil and pour in the egg mixture. Sprinkle over the remaining feta before placing in the oven.

8 Place in the oven and bake for 40 minutes to 1 hour. Keep checking the middle with a knife (it should come out dry).

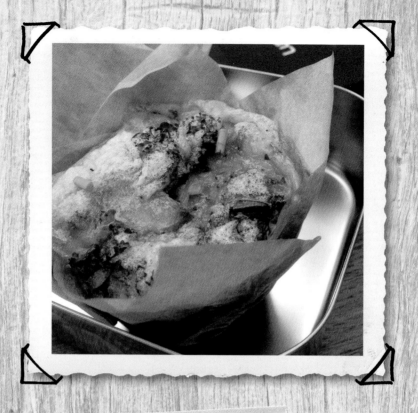

Omegas To Go Muffins

Ingredients
★ 6 eggs
★ ½ tsp baking soda
★ 3.5 oz (100g) smoked salmon, chopped
★ 1 handful kale, chopped

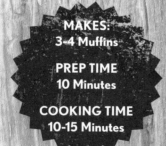

MAKES:
3-4 Muffins

PREP TIME
10 Minutes

COOKING TIME
10-15 Minutes

1 Preheat the oven to 350°F.

2 Grease a muffin pan with a little coconut oil or olive oil to prevent the muffins from sticking.

3 Beat the eggs and baking soda in a bowl or using a blender or food processor.

4 Stir in the kale and salmon and mix well.

5 Pour the mixture into the prepared muffin pan and place in the oven to cook for 10-15 minutes.

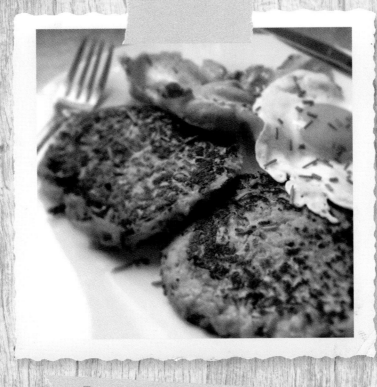

Sweet Potato Hash Browns

Ingredients

★ 4 medium sweet potatoes
★ 1 egg, beaten
★ 4 scallions, thinly chopped
★ 5 tbsp (80g) ground almonds
   (or you can substitute rice flour)
★ Himalayan Pink salt
★ Freshly ground black pepper
★ 2 tbsp coconut oil, olive oil or butter
   for cooking

MAKES:
6 Hash Browns

PREP TIME
8 Minutes

COOKING TIME
8-10 Minutes

1 Peel and steam two of the sweet potatoes. While they cook, peel and grate the other two and place them in a bowl with the scallions, ground almonds, salt, pepper and beaten egg.

2 Once the sweet potato is soft right through, add it to the other ingredients and mash them all together.

3 Heat the oil in a pan and form the mix into patties. Don't make them too thick, otherwise they won't cook through. Add them to the pan to cook.

4 Flatten in the pan with a spatula and cook for 4 minutes on each side or until golden and crispy.

5 Serve with eggs for breakfast or your protein of choice at dinner time.

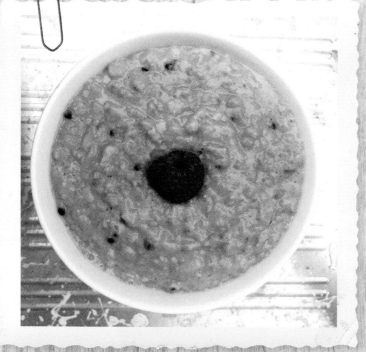

Raspberry and Apple Power Oatmeal

Ingredients

★ ¼ cup (100g) of gluten free oats
   (substitute rice flakes, buckwheat or
   quinoa and follow the cooking
   guidance if different from steps
   outlined)
★ 2 cups (500 ml) unsweetened
   almond milk or unsweetened
   coconut milk
★ 1 medium apple, grated
★ 3.5 oz (100g) raspberries
★ ½ tsp cinnamon
★ Pinch of nutmeg
★ 2-3 tsp raw honey or xylitol (optional)
★ 3 tbsp (40g) protein powder

1 Place the oats in a saucepan and top with the milk. Stir in the apple and raspberries and place on a medium heat.

2 Simmer for 5-10 minutes, stirring occasionally.

3 Remove from the heat and stir in the spices, protein powder and top with a drizzle of honey or xylitol.

TIP

Soak the oats with the milk, apple and raspberries in the fridge overnight to improve taste and digestibility.

You can make this with goat's, sheep's or cow's milk if tolerated and omit the protein powder.

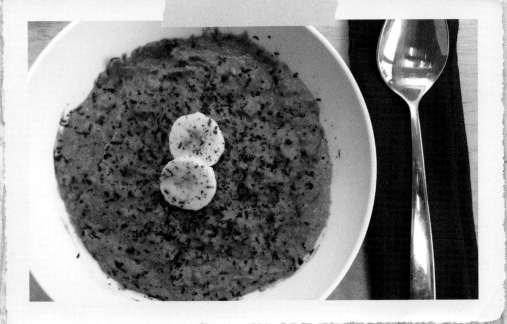

Chocolate
Ready Brekkie

Ingredients

★ 2 ripe bananas
★ 4 tsp (20g) chocolate protein powder
★ ⅔ cup (150 ml) almond milk
★ 1 egg
★ 1 tbsp almond butter
★ Pinch of Celtic Sea or Himalayan Pink salt
★ 1 tsp coconut oil

OPTIONAL

★ 1 square dark chocolate

1 Blend all the ingredients, except for the coconut oil, in a food processor or blender to mix it all together. Be careful not to blend for too long.

2 Heat the coconut oil in a pan over a medium heat and add the mixture. Keep an eye on it and stir occasionally until it reaches the thickness you desire.

3 Top with a little grated dark chocolate and enjoy.

SERVES: 1

PREP TIME
3 Minutes

COOKING TIME
3-5 Minutes

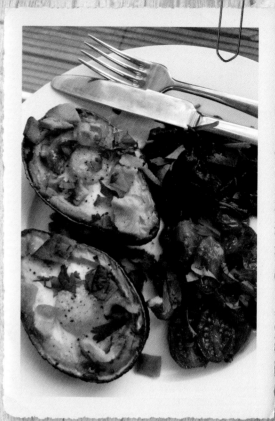

SERVES: 1

PREP TIME
5 Minutes

COOKING TIME
10-15 Minutes
(or microwave
for 8 minutes)

Eggs in
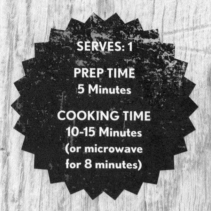

Avo Boats
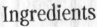

Ingredients
★ 1 medium or large avocado
★ 2 small eggs
★ Pinch of Celtic Sea or Himalayan Pink
   salt and freshly ground black pepper
★ Sprinkle of garlic powder
★ 1 tbsp coconut oil
★ 1-2 strips of bacon
★ 1 handful cherry tomatoes
★ 1 handful spinach
★ Fresh cilantro

1 Preheat the oven to 350°F.

2 Halve the avocado, remove the stone and slice a little off the bottom so each half will lay flat on a baking tray.

3 Remove a little more avocado flesh to ensure there is enough room for the egg.

4 Add one egg to each half and top with the salt, pepper and garlic before placing on a baking tray in the oven for 10-15 minutes.

5 When the eggs are around 5 minutes from being cooked, heat the coconut oil in a frying pan over a medium heat and add the bacon and tomatoes. Cook until the bacon starts to brown and the tomatoes soften. Add the spinach and sauté.

6 Ensure the eggs are fully cooked before serving with the spinach and tomatoes. Chop the bacon and fresh cilantro and sprinkle over the top.

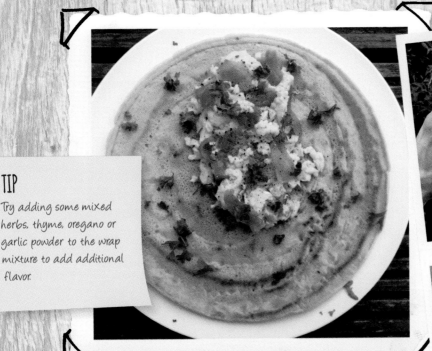

Fitter Breakfast Wraps

Ingredients

★ 4 eggs
★ 2 cups (475 ml) unsweetened almond or coconut milk (carton based, not canned)
★ 1 cup (245g) tapioca flour
★ 4 tbsp (60g) coconut flour
★ Pinch of Celtic Sea or Himalayan Pink salt and freshly ground black pepper

SUGGESTED FILLINGS

★ Smoked salmon
★ Avocado
★ Eggs
★ Bacon

MAKES:
6-8 Wraps

PREP TIME
3 Minutes

COOKING TIME
2-4 Minutes
per wrap

1 Beat the eggs in a bowl and add the tapioca, coconut flour, salt and pepper, and beat again thoroughly until the mixture is a smooth batter.

2 Heat a non-stick pan over a medium heat.

3 Using a large serving spoon, pour around ¼ of the batter into the center of the pan. Tip the pan from side to side to allow the batter to run to the edge of the pan and cover the entire base.

4 Cook for 1-2 minutes before flipping and cook the underside until golden. Repeat three more times with the remaining batter.

5 You can make smaller wraps with a smaller frying pan.

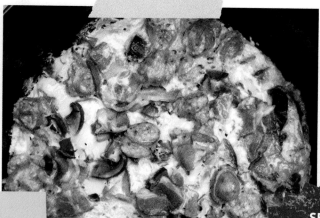

SERVES: 6

PREP TIME
20 Minutes

SLOW COOKING TIME
low heat 6-8 hours
or 4 hours on high

Big Breakfast ZZZ Bake

Ingredients

★ 1 lb (500g) of chopped sweet potato or new potatoes
★ 6 gluten-free sausages, chopped into small pieces
★ 7 slices of bacon, chopped into small pieces
★ 1 large red onion, chopped
★ 1 large handful of spinach
★ 4 scallions, chopped
★ 1 large carrot, sliced with a julienne peeler
★ 1-¾ cup (400 ml) goat's milk (for a dairy free alternative substitute canned coconut milk)
★ 10 eggs
★ 1 tbsp of mixed herbs
★ Celtic Sea or Himalayan Pink salt and freshly ground black pepper

No-fuss version of a full English breakfast that cooks overnight.

1 Grease the inside of the slow cooker with butter, ghee or coconut oil.

2 Place the potatoes on the bottom of the pot.

3 Layer half of the sausage, bacon and red onion on top of the potatoes and sprinkle with half the mixed herbs.

4 Place the spinach on top to form a new layer.

5 Add the grated carrot and chopped scallions to form the next layer.

6 Then add the remaining chopped meat, onion and herbs to finish.

7 Blend the eggs with the milk and pour over the contents of the slow cooker pot.

8 Set your slow cooker to a low setting and cook overnight for 6-8 hours.

9 Catch yourself some zzz, then wake up and enjoy.

SERVES: 2

PREP TIME
5 Minutes

COOKING TIME
12 Minutes

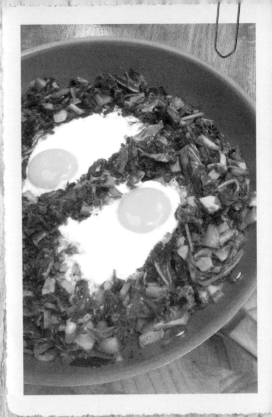

One Pan Breakfast

Ingredients

★ 2 tbsp coconut oil, olive oil or butter for cooking
★ 2 cloves garlic, peeled and finely chopped
★ 1-2 handfuls of cooked potatoes, chopped into small chunks
★ 4 slices of bacon, chopped
★ 1 handful mushrooms, sliced
★ 2 handfuls cherry tomatoes, chopped
★ 1 large handful kale, chopped,
★ 1 large handful spinach
★ 2 tsp smoked paprika
★ ½ tsp cayenne pepper powder (optional)
★ Celtic Sea or Himalayan Pink salt and freshly ground black pepper
★ 4 eggs

This is a great recipe to use up leftovers, and the quantity depends on how many people you're cooking for.

1 Heat the oil in a pan over a medium heat before adding the garlic, chopped potatoes, bacon, mushrooms and cherry tomatoes, and cook for about 5 minutes or until the potatoes turn golden.

2 Add the kale, spinach, paprika, salt and pepper, and stir well. Cook for another 4-5 minutes until the kale and spinach have wilted down.

3 Create four holes in the mixture and crack an egg into each one. Continue to cook until the eggs are completely cooked.

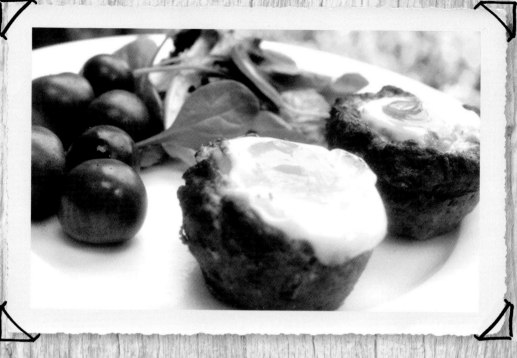

Piggy Pots

Ingredients

- ★ 1 lb (500g) ground pork
- ★ 2 tsp smoked paprika
- ★ ½-1 tsp chili powder
- ★ 1 tsp onion powder
- ★ ½ tsp garlic powder
- ★ 1 tbsp tomato purée
- ★ Celtic Sea or Himalayan Pink salt and freshly ground black pepper
- ★ 6 eggs
- ★ Fresh cilantro to serve

SERVES: 6

PREP TIME
10 Minutes

COOKING TIME
20-25 Minutes

1 Preheat the oven to 350°F.

2 Using your hands, thoroughly mix all the ingredients except the eggs and cilantro in a bowl.

3 Place a small handful of the mixture into a muffin pan and pat the meat flat. Using your finger, mold it into the side of the pan to make an egg cup. Ideally the meat mixture should be ⅓ inch (1 cm) higher than the top of the pan. If the pork layer is too thick there won't be enough room for the egg.

4 Make six cups in the mixture and then add an egg to each one before placing in the oven to cook for 20-25 minutes or until the egg has fully cooked.

5 Top with fresh cilantro to serve.

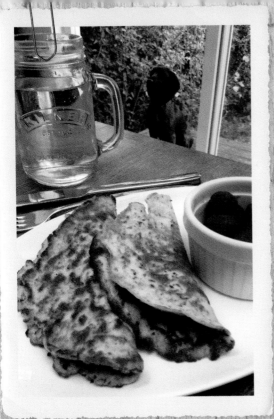

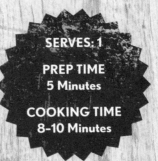
Cottage Flaxcakes

Ingredients

★ 3 eggs
★ 3 heaped tbsp cottage cheese
★ 1 tbsp flaxseed
★ Butter or olive oil for cooking

TO SERVE
★ Fresh berries and cinnamon

1 Place a knob of butter or a splash of olive oil in a non-stick frying pan over a moderate heat.

2 Beat the eggs and cottage cheese in a bowl until combined.

3 Stir in the flaxseed.

4 Gently pour the mixture into the pan and cook for 4-5 minutes before flipping over to cook the underside.

5 Serve with fresh berries and a sprinkle of cinnamon.

TIP

Smaller flaxcakes are easier to flip!

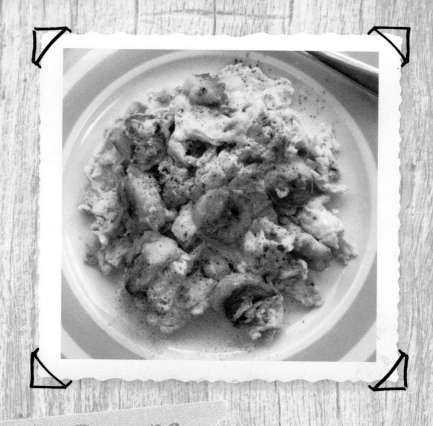

Salty Banana Cinnamon Scramble

Ingredients

★ 2-3 eggs
★ 1 banana, sliced
★ Coconut oil for cooking
★ A sprinkle of cinnamon
★ A sprinkle of Himalayan Pink or Celtic Sea salt
★ Salad to serve

1 Place the coconut oil in a pan and melt over a low heat.

2 Add the sliced banana to the pan and cook gently for 5 minutes, flipping occasionally.

3 Beat the eggs in a bowl and add to the pan. Toss the banana and eggs with a spatula, allowing the eggs to scramble.

4 Top the eggs and banana with cinnamon and salt, and serve with a large salad.

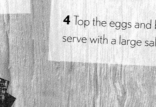

SERVES: 1

PREP TIME
3 Minutes

COOKING TIME
5 Minutes

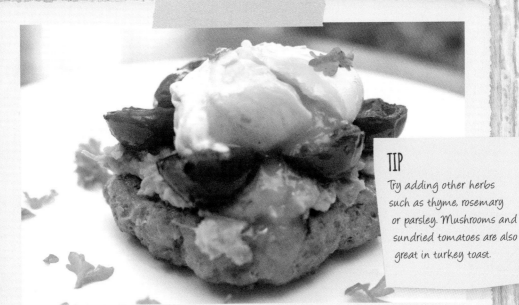

TIP

Try adding other herbs such as thyme, rosemary or parsley. Mushrooms and sundried tomatoes are also great in turkey toast.

Turkey Toast Toppers

Ingredients

★ 1 lb (500g) ground turkey thigh (ground breast is fine but has a little drier texture)
★ 1 tsp mixed herbs
★ 1 tbsp olive oil or butter for cooking
★ 1 avocado, peeled and mashed
★ 1 handful cherry tomatoes, halved
★ 4 eggs
★ Salt and pepper
★ 1 tbsp fresh parsley (to serve)

SERVES: 4

PREP TIME
4 Minutes

COOKING TIME
10–12 Minutes

1 Heat the oil in a frying pan over a low heat.

2 Mix the turkey and herbs together in a bowl using your hands. Season with salt and pepper.

3 There are two ways to make these into slices of toast. Either: flatten the turkey mixture onto a sheet of parchment paper and then cut into squares using a sharp knife. Use a spatula to scoop up each square and place in the pan. Alternatively you can simply flatten out the turkey mixture onto a sheet of parchment paper and then place into the pan as one large square, cutting into smaller squares while in the pan.

4 Cook for around 10 minutes, flipping each one over after 5 minutes. Ideally they should be golden brown on both sides and fully cooked.

5 While the turkey toast is cooking, bring a pan of water to a boil and gently poach the eggs. Time them so they are ready at the same time as the toast. Heat a little oil in a frying pan and sauté the cherry tomatoes until soft.

6 Once the turkey is fully cooked, remove from the pan. Spread over a thin layer of mashed avocado and top with an egg and a spoonful of the cooked cherry tomatoes. Serve sprinkled with fresh parsley.

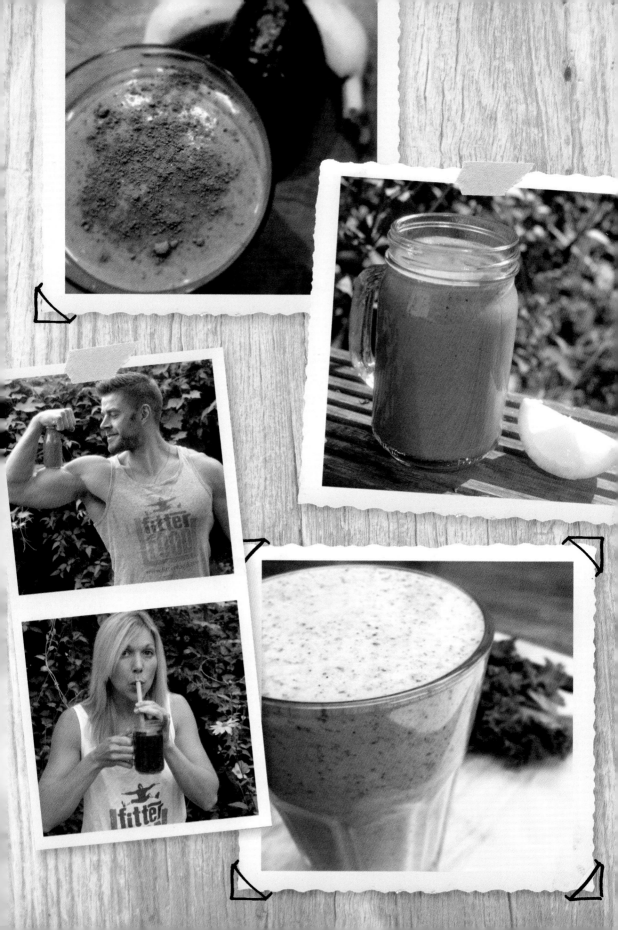

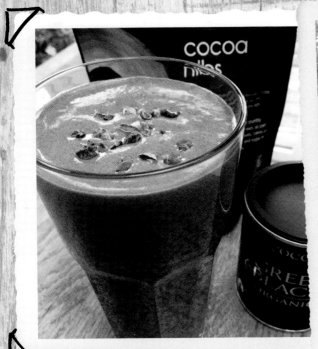

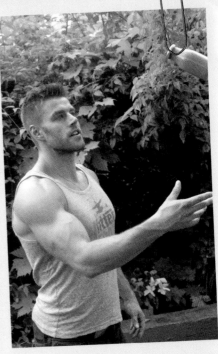

2

Protein Smoothies

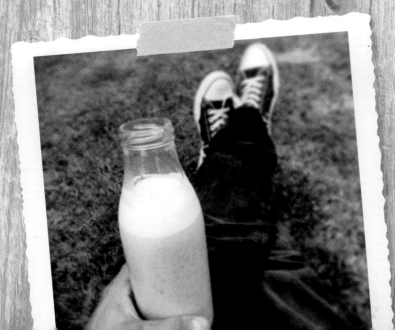

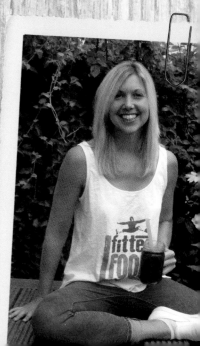

How to Make the Perfect Smoothie

We love smoothies, but many people make the mistake of including too much fruit and not enough protein, fats and fiber to keep blood sugar stable and hunger at bay.

The following easy, step-by-step guide illustrates how to put together a smashing smoothie:

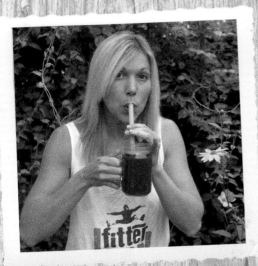

STEP 1

ADD ½ to ¾ OUNCES (15-25G) PROTEIN

- ✔ whey
- ✔ rice
- ✔ hemp
- ✔ pea
- ✔ collagen
- ✔ eggs

STEP 2

ADD A SERVING OF FAT

- ✔ ½ small avocado
- ✔ egg yolks
- ✔ 1 tbsp nut butter
- ✔ 10-12 nuts
- ✔ 1 tbsp butter or ghee
- ✔ 1 tbsp seeds (flax, chia, hemp or pumpkin)
- ✔ coconut oil, coconut milk or coconut cream

STEP 3

ADD 1-2 SERVINGS OF ANY FRUIT (OPTIONAL)

- ✔ fresh or frozen berries
- ✔ banana
- ✔ kiwi
- ✔ melon
- ✔ apple
- ✔ pear
- ✔ peach
- ✔ plum
- ✔ pineapple
- ✔ mango

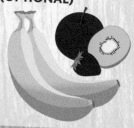

STEP 4

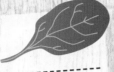

ADD 1-2 SERVINGS OF GREENS

- ✔ spinach
- ✔ kale
- ✔ lettuce
- ✔ watercress

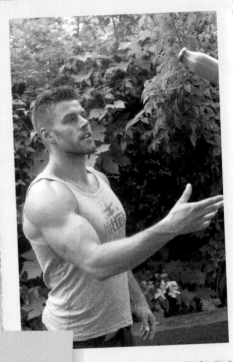

STEP 5

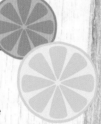

ADD MIXERS

- ✔ water
- ✔ fresh lime or lemon juice
- ✔ coconut water
- ✔ unsweetened coconut milk
- ✔ unsweetened almond milk

TIP

Keep your fruit, milks and water mixers chilled before blending, as the cooler the smoothie the nicer the taste!

STEP 6

SWEETEN TO TASTE (OPTIONAL)

- ✔ 1-2 tsp raw, unpasteurized honey
- ✔ Sweet Drops Stevia Clear by Sweetleaf
- ✔ Xylitol
- ✔ 1-2 medjool dates
- ✔ 2-3 dried apricots

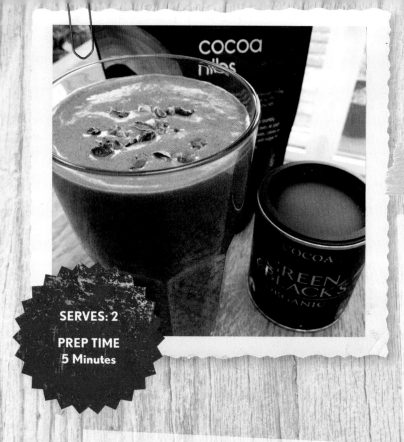

Mint Choc Chip

Ingredients

★ 4 tsp (20g) protein powder
★ 1 banana
★ 1 handful spinach
★ 4 tsp (2 dsp) cacao/cocoa powder
★ 3-4 drops peppermint extract (more if you like it minty)
★ 2 tsp Xylitol or raw honey
★ 1 cup (250 ml) unsweetened almond milk
★ Cacao nibs to sprinkle on top (optional)

SERVES: 2

PREP TIME
5 Minutes

TO MAKE BOTH SMOOTHIES
Place all the ingredients in a blender and mix until smooth.
Add a little more water if needed for the desired consistency.

Choc Avo Bliss

Ingredients

★ 1 avocado
★ 4 tsp (20g) protein powder
★ 2 frozen bananas
★ 1 handful mixed berries
★ 2 tbsp cocoa powder
★ 2 cups (500 ml) unsweetened almond or coconut milk

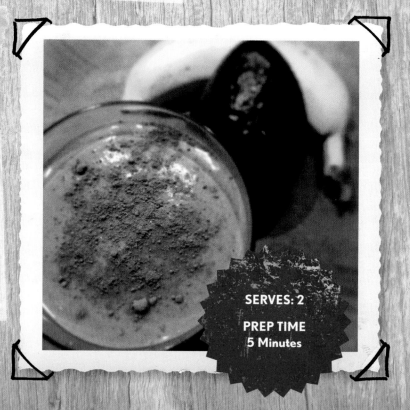

SERVES: 2

PREP TIME
5 Minutes

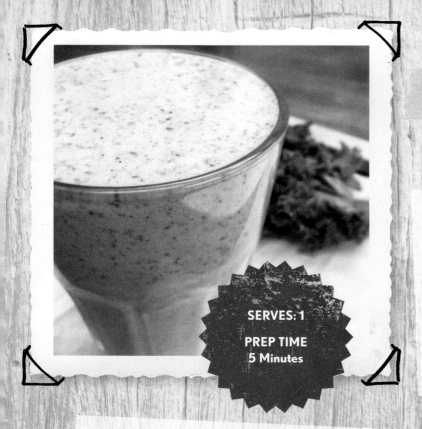

Hidden Greens

Ingredients

★ 4 tsp (20g) protein powder
★ 1 kiwi, peeled
★ 1 handful strawberries
★ 1 handful kale
★ 1 handful watercress
★ 1 tbsp cashew butter
★ 2 tbsp broccoli sprouts (optional)
★ 1 cup (250 ml) unsweetened almond milk

SERVES: 1

PREP TIME
5 Minutes

TO MAKE BOTH SMOOTHIES
Place all the ingredients in a blender and mix until smooth.
Add a little more water if needed for the desired consistency.

SERVES: 1–2

PREP TIME
5 Minutes

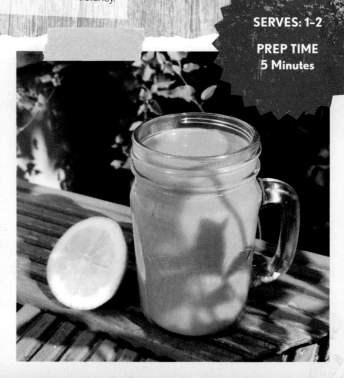

Carrot and Mango

Ingredients

★ 4 tsp (20g) protein powder
★ 1 mango (peeled and stone removed)
★ 2 medium carrots
★ ⅔ cup (150 ml) canned coconut milk
★ A squeeze of fresh lemon juice
★ ⅔ cup (150 ml) water

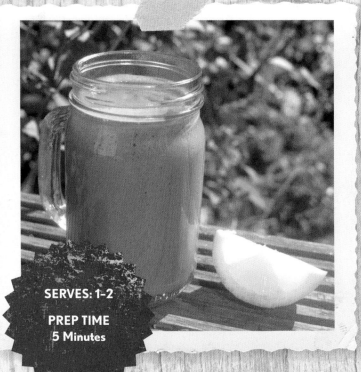

Ingredients

★ 4 tsp (20g) vanilla protein powder
★ 1 small pear (core removed)
★ 1 handful spinach
★ 1 handful kale
★ 1 tbsp almond butter
★ 1 cup (250 ml) unsweetened almond milk

SERVES: 1-2

PREP TIME
5 Minutes

TO MAKE BOTH SMOOTHIES
Place all the ingredients in a blender and mix until smooth.
Add a little more water if needed for the desired consistency.

Banana Bread

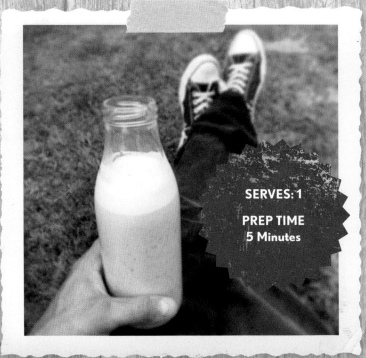

Ingredients

★ 4 tsp (20g) protein powder
★ 1 banana
★ 1 tbsp cashew butter
★ 1 tbsp chia or flaxseed
★ 1 tsp vanilla extract
★ ½ tsp cinnamon
★ 1 cup (250 ml) unsweetened coconut (carton based) or almond milk

SERVES: 1

PREP TIME
5 Minutes

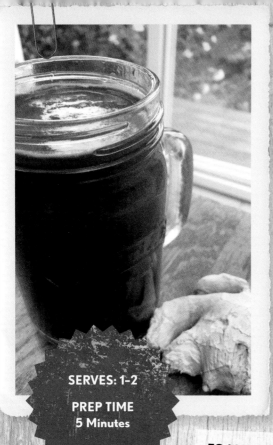

Kale Chocolate Ginger

Ingredients

★ 4 tsp (20g) vanilla protein powder
★ 2 tbsp cacao/cocoa powder
★ 1 large chunk of fresh ginger or
   1 tsp ginger powder
★ 1 handful kale
★ 1 banana
★ 2-3 tsp Xylitol or 1 tsp raw honey
★ 1 cup (250 ml) unsweetened
   almond milk

SERVES: 1-2

PREP TIME
5 Minutes

TO MAKE BOTH SMOOTHIES
Place all the ingredients in a blender and mix until smooth.
Add a little more water if needed for the desired consistency.

Coconut Greens

Ingredients

★ 4 tsp (20g) vanilla protein
   powder
★ ½ cup (100 ml) canned
   coconut milk
★ 1 handful frozen raspberries
★ Juice of half a lime
★ 1 handful kale or spinach
★ 1 tsp Xylitol or raw honey
★ 1 cup (250 ml) water

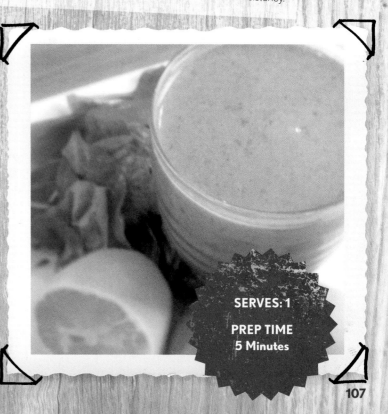

SERVES: 1

PREP TIME
5 Minutes

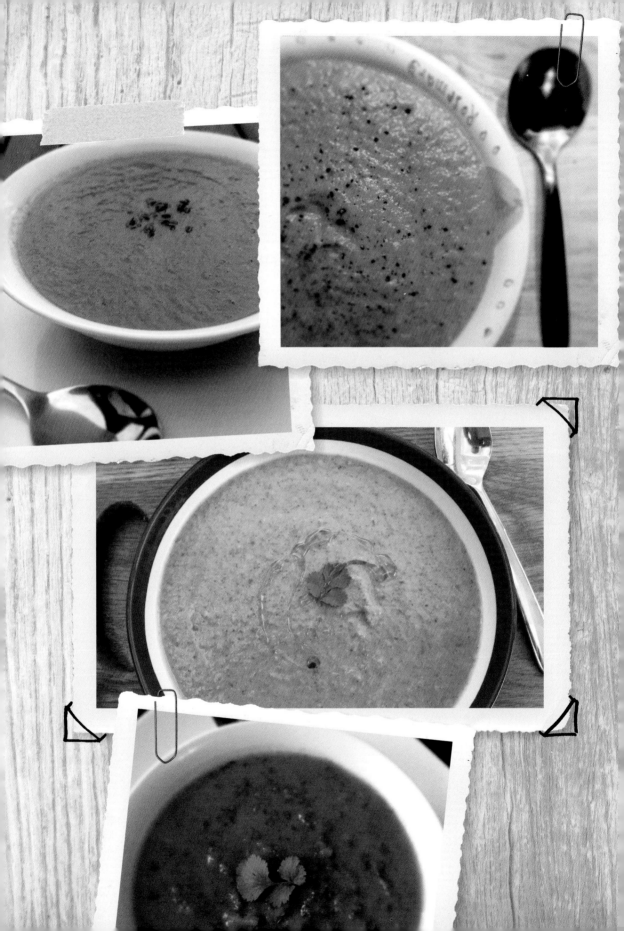

3 Soups

Make your soups with homemade bone broth for an extra dose of minerals and essential proteins. See page 209.

Carrot and Apple Soup

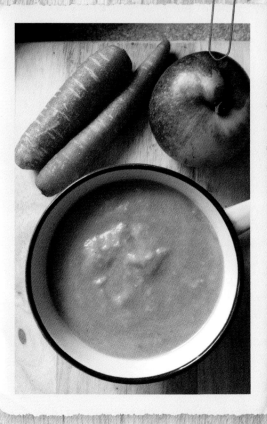

Ingredients

★ 2 tbsp olive oil
★ 2 apples, chopped, cores removed
★ 1 leek, chopped
★ 5 large carrots, chopped
★ 2 inch chunk of ginger, peeled and finely chopped
★ 1 can coconut milk
★ 1 cup (250 ml) bone broth/stock or water (add extra for a thinner soup)
★ ½ tsp Himalayan Pink salt
★ Freshly ground black pepper

1 Heat the olive oil in a pan and sauté the leek, carrot and apple until tender. Add the fresh ginger, coconut milk and broth/stock or water.

2 Cook for 25-30 minutes until the carrots are soft. Purée using a hand blender or food processor. Once cooked, season with salt and pepper to your taste.

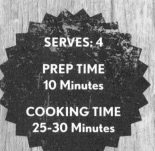

SERVES: 4

PREP TIME
10 Minutes

COOKING TIME
25-30 Minutes

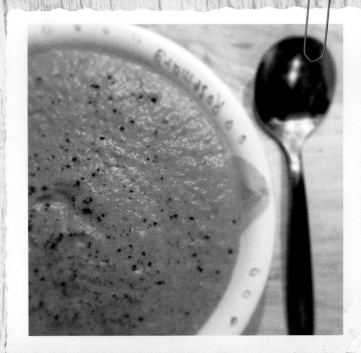

SERVES: 8

PREP TIME
10 Minutes

COOKING TIME
25 Minutes

Hulk Soup

Ingredients

★ 2 tbsp coconut oil
★ 4 cloves garlic, finely chopped
★ 2 dice-sized cubes of fresh ginger, peeled and finely chopped
★ 1 onion, peeled and chopped
★ 4 leeks, chopped
★ 1-⅓ lbs (600g) frozen peas
★ 4 zucchini, chopped
★ 1 whole head of broccoli, chopped
★ ½ lb (250g) green beans, chopped
★ 1 handful fresh mint
★ 3-¼ cups (800 ml) bone broth/stock or vegetable stock
★ Himalayan Pink salt and freshly ground black pepper to taste
★ 1 large bag of spinach
★ 4 heaped tbsp green pesto

1 Heat the coconut oil in a large saucepan and then add the garlic, ginger, onion and leeks, and cook for a couple of minutes, stirring occasionally.

2 Now add the peas, zucchini, broccoli, green beans and mint and stir a little before adding the broth/stock, salt and pepper. Bring to a boil and leave to simmer for 25 minutes or until the vegetables are cooked, stirring through occasionally. The broth/stock should just cover all the vegetables.

3 Add the bag of spinach and stir in to wilt down before using a stick blender or food processor to mix the ingredients together. Taste and add more salt and pepper if required. If too thick, add some more stock or water.

4 Stir in the pesto, taste again and serve.

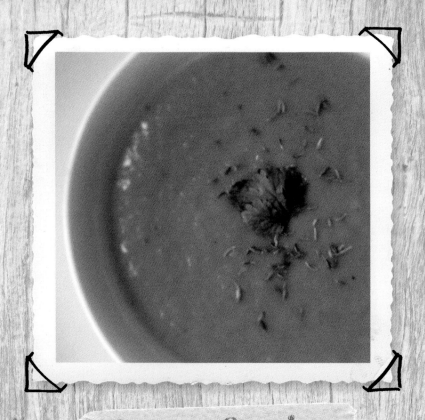

Carrot, Cumin and Ginger Soup

Ingredients

★ 1 tbsp coconut oil, butter or olive oil for cooking
★ 2 cloves garlic, peeled and finely chopped
★ 1-inch chunk of ginger, peeled and finely chopped
★ 2-¼ lbs (1 kg) carrots, roughly chopped
★ 2 tsp ground cumin
★ 4-¼ cups (1 liter) bone broth/stock
★ Himalayan Pink or Celtic Sea salt and black pepper to taste
★ 1 tbsp cumin seeds to sprinkle

1 Sauté the garlic and ginger in the coconut oil for 2-3 minutes.

2 Add the carrots and cook for around 5 minutes.

3 Add the broth/stock and cumin powder and simmer for about 45 minutes to 1 hour until the carrot is soft.

4 Season with salt and pepper to taste.

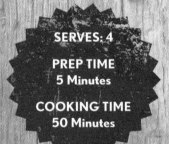

SERVES: 4

PREP TIME
5 Minutes

COOKING TIME
50 Minutes

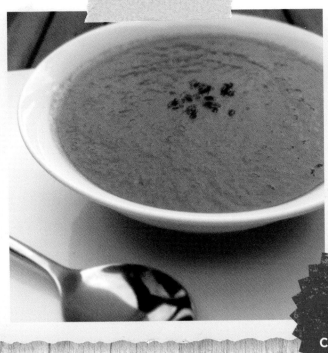

SERVES: 6

PREP TIME
4 Minutes

COOKING TIME
15 Minutes

Chili Chicken and Tomato Soup

Ingredients

★ 2 tbsp coconut oil, butter or olive oil for cooking
★ 1 red onion, peeled and chopped
★ 3 red bell peppers, chopped
★ 1 red chili, finely chopped
★ 3 cloves garlic, crushed
★ 2-3 sprigs fresh thyme
★ 2-1/3 cups 650 ml chicken bone broth/stock
★ 14 ounces (400g) can chopped tomatoes
★ 1 heaped tsp smoked paprika
★ Himalayan Pink salt and freshly ground black pepper

1 Add the coconut oil to a large saucepan over a medium heat, then add the onion, peppers, chili, garlic, thyme, salt and pepper. Stir well and cook for about 4-5 minutes.

2 Once the vegetables start to soften, add the chicken broth/stock, chopped tomatoes and smoked paprika and stir well.

3 Bring to a boil and then simmer for about 10 minutes.

4 Once cooked, use a stick blender to mix thoroughly.

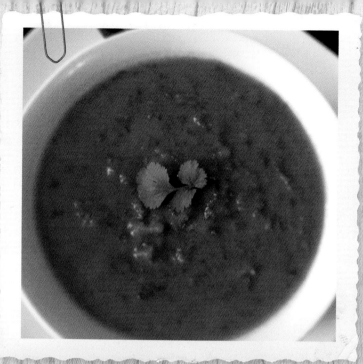

SERVES: 6

PREP TIME
10 Minutes

COOKING TIME
50 Minutes

Sweet Potato and Kale Soup

Ingredients

★ 1 onion, chopped
★ 2 large sweet potatoes, peeled and cut into small cubes
★ 1 carton chopped tomatoes
★ 3 cloves garlic, crushed or finely chopped
★ 1 tbsp curry powder
★ ¼ tsp garam masala
★ ½ tsp cumin
★ 2 cups (500 ml) broth/stock
★ 1 cup (250 ml) water
★ 1 bunch kale, coarsely chopped

1 Place the onion, sweet potato, tomatoes, garlic and spices in a saucepan. Cover with the broth/stock and water.

2 Simmer over a low heat for around 40 minutes or until all the vegetables are cooked.

3 Add the kale and cook for another 10 minutes. Use a hand blender or food processor to blend.

114

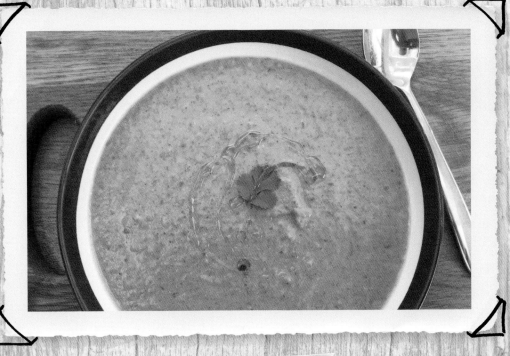

Creamy Broccoli, Kale and Ginger Soup

SERVES: 6

PREP TIME
10 Minutes

COOKING TIME
20-25 Minutes

Ingredients

★ 2 tbsp coconut oil, butter or olive oil for cooking
★ 1 onion, chopped
★ 3 cloves garlic, peeled and finely chopped
★ 5 inches ginger, peeled and finely chopped
★ 1-½ pounds (700g) broccoli (split into small florets)
★ 1 large handful kale, roughly chopped
★ 1 large handful fresh cilantro, roughly chopped
★ Celtic Sea or Himalayan Pink salt and freshly ground black pepper
★ 2 cups (500 ml) coconut milk
★ 3-¼ cups (800 ml) broth/stock or vegetable stock (depending on the desired consistency)
★ Cilantro to garnish

1 Heat the coconut oil in a large saucepan over a medium heat and add the onion, garlic and ginger, and stir. Cook for around 5 minutes until the onion softens.

2 Add the broccoli, kale and cilantro, and stir well again. Cook for a few minutes before adding the coconut milk and broth/stock. Bring to a boil and then simmer for around 15 minutes or until the broccoli is soft.

3 Use a hand blender or food processor to blend. If the soup is too thick, simply add a little leftover stock or water.

4 Season to taste and top with fresh cilantro and a drizzle of olive oil .

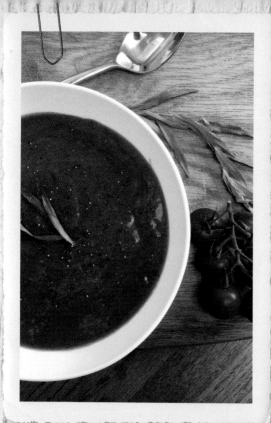

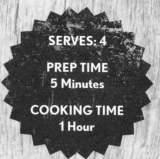

SERVES: 4

PREP TIME
5 Minutes

COOKING TIME
1 Hour

Tomato and Tarragon Soup

Ingredients
★ 1-⅔ pounds (750g) cherry tomatoes
★ 2 red peppers, chopped
★ 3 cloves garlic, peeled
★ 3 tbsp olive oil
★ Celtic Sea or Himalayan Pink salt
   and freshly ground black pepper
★ 1 handful fresh tarragon
★ 4-¼ cups (1 liter) broth/stock or
   vegetable stock

1 Preheat the oven to 350°F.

2 Place the tomatoes and peppers in a baking tray and toss in the garlic, olive oil and seasoning before putting in the oven to cook for 45 minutes, stirring occasionally.

3 Once cooked, heat the stock and fresh tarragon in a large saucepan.

4 Add the baked tomatoes and peppers to the broth/stock and bring to a simmer.

5 Use a stick blender or food processor to blend.

6 Season to taste and serve.

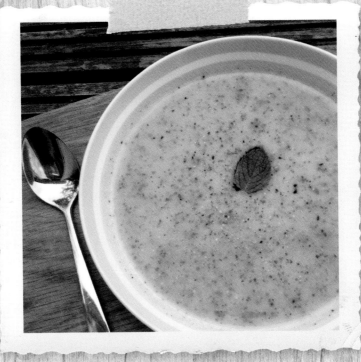

Minty Zucchini Soup

Ingredients

★ 2 tbsp olive oil
★ 1 onion, peeled and chopped
★ 2 cloves garlic, peeled and chopped
★ 3 zucchini, chopped
★ 4-¼ cups (1 liter) broth/stock or vegetable stock
★ 1 handful fresh mint, roughly chopped
★ Celtic Sea or Himalayan Pink salt and freshly ground black pepper

1 Heat the oil in a large saucepan over a medium heat before adding the onion and garlic and cooking for 5 minutes until soft.

2 Add the zucchini and cook for another 5 minutes, stirring occasionally.

3 Add the broth/stock, fresh mint, salt and pepper, and simmer for about 5 minutes.

4 Using a hand blender or food processor, blend the ingredients to your desired consistency.

SERVES: 6

PREP TIME
5 Minutes

COOKING TIME
15 Minutes

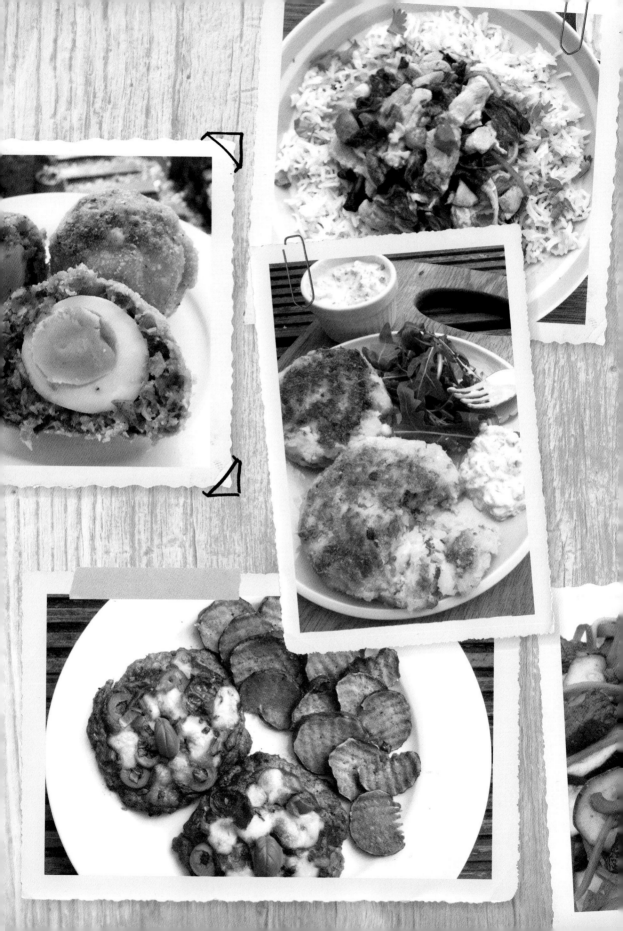

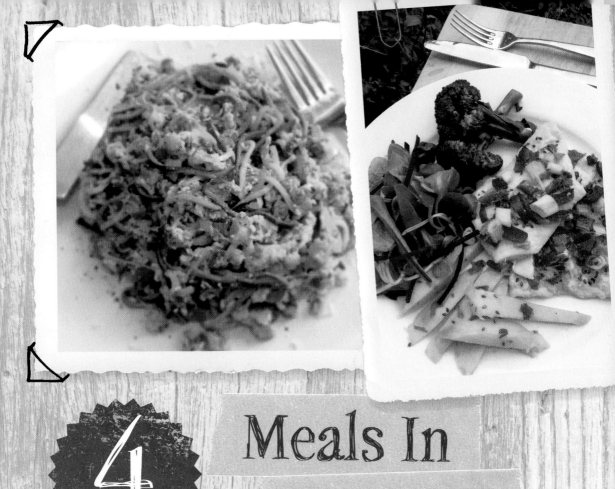

4 Meals In Minutes

Fish

Poultry

Meat

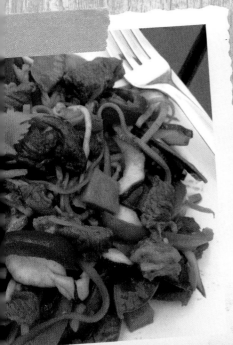

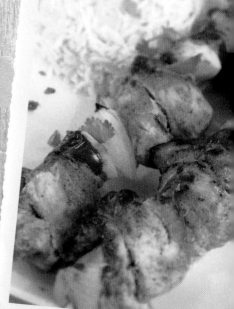

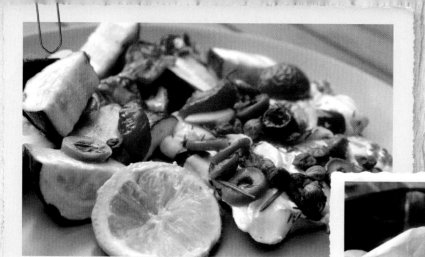

Fish in a Mediterranean Bag

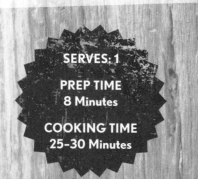

Ingredients

★ 1 large fillet white fish
★ 1 zucchini, sliced
★ 6 cherry tomatoes, halved
★ 1 tbsp capers
★ 5 olives, thinly sliced
★ 1 sprig of fresh rosemary, chopped
★ 3-4 fresh basil leaves, torn
★ 2-3 slices of lemon
★ Himalayan Pink or Celtic Sea salt
    and pepper to taste
★ Olive oil

SERVES: 1

PREP TIME
8 Minutes

COOKING TIME
25-30 Minutes

1 Preheat the oven to 350°F

2 Lay out a sheet of parchment paper and place your fish in the center.

3 Scatter the zucchini and cherry tomatoes around the edge of the fish.

4 Top the fish and vegetables with the capers, sliced olives, rosemary and basil.

5 Place the lemon slices on top and season with salt and pepper.

6 Drizzle olive oil over the fish and vegetables.

7 Take the four corners of the parchment paper and gather together, twisting the paper to seal the fish and vegetables inside. Place on a baking tray.

8 Place in the oven to cook. Check the fish after 25-30 minutes. The tomatoes should be soft and the fish fully cooked.

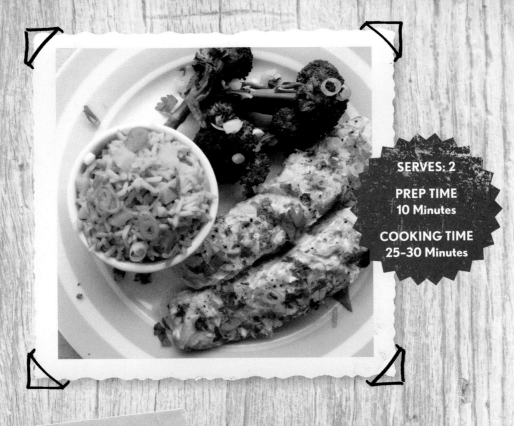

SERVES: 2

PREP TIME
10 Minutes

COOKING TIME
25–30 Minutes

Fish in a Caribbean Bag

Ingredients

★ 2 salmon fillets
★ Zest and juice of 1 lemon
★ 2 scallions, chopped
★ 2 cloves garlic, peeled and finely chopped
★ 1 dice-sized chunk of ginger, peeled and chopped
★ 1 tsp crushed chilies OR ½ Scotch bonnet chili, deseeded and chopped
★ Celtic Sea or Himalayan Pink salt and freshly ground black pepper
★ 2 tbsp fresh cilantro

1 Preheat the oven to 350°F.

2 Lay a sheet of parchment paper on a baking dish and place the fish in the center.

3 Scatter over the lemon zest and juice, scallions, garlic, ginger, Scotch bonnet or crushed chilies, fresh cilantro and seasoning.

4 Take the four corners of the parchment paper and gather together, twisting the paper to seal the fish and vegetables inside.

5 Place in the oven to cook. Check the fish after 20-25 minutes. Serve once fully cooked.

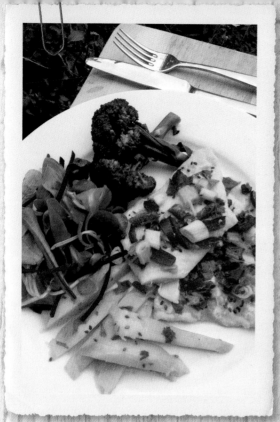

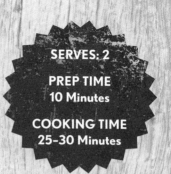

Fish in a Thai Bag

Ingredients

★ 2 white fish fillets
★ ½ cup (100 ml) coconut milk
★ 1 red pepper, deseeded and chopped
★ 2 scallions, chopped
★ Juice and zest of 1 lime
★ 1 clove garlic, peeled and finely
  chopped
★ 1 dice-sized chunk of ginger, peeled
  and grated
★ 1 tbsp tamari
★ 1 tsp fish sauce (optional)

TO SERVE
★ Fresh cilantro (optional)

1 Preheat the oven to 350°F.

2 Lay a sheet of parchment paper on a baking dish and place the fish in the center.

3 Scatter over the pepper and scallions.

4 In a bowl, mix the coconut milk, lime zest and juice, garlic, ginger, tamari and fish sauce.

5 Pour the coconut milk mixture over the fish.

6 Take the four corners of the parchment paper and gather together, twisting the paper to seal the fish and vegetables inside.

7 Place in the oven to cook. Check the fish after 20-25 minutes. Serve once fully cooked.

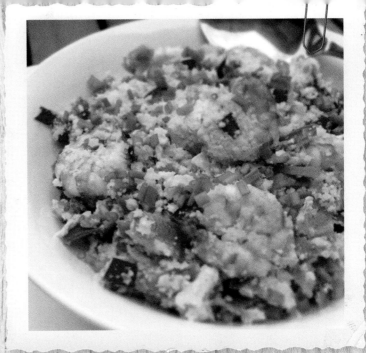

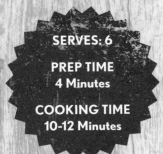

Stir Fried Shrimp
with Cauliflower Rice

Ingredients

★ 1 tbsp coconut oil
★ 1-¾ pound (800g) shrimp
★ 1 red onion, peeled and diced
★ 5 scallions, finely chopped
★ 1 red bell pepper, diced
★ 1 green bell pepper, diced
★ 2 cloves of garlic, crushed or finely chopped
★ 1 large carrot, peeled and diced
★ 3 tbsp tamari, or if you can get it, coconut aminos
★ 1 tbsp toasted sesame oil
★ 4-5 drops fish sauce
★ 3 eggs, beaten
★ 1 large cauliflower
★ 1 large handful fresh chives, chopped
★ Celtic Sea or Himalayan Pink salt

1 Before you start, get your cauliflower rice ready. Simply use a grater to grate the florets of cauliflower into a bowl. Don't press too hard as you won't get the rice-like consistency. Or if you have a blender, just use that. It won't take long.

2 Heat the coconut oil in a wok or a large pan and then add the peppers, onion, scallions, carrot and garlic. Stir to coat in the oil and sauté them for about 4 minutes, stirring occasionally.

3 Now add the shrimp and salt, and stir well again. Once they start to turn pink, add the tamari and toasted sesame oil, and stir well again. Cook for about 2 minutes.

4 Add the egg to the pan, and as it starts to set add the cauliflower rice and give it another good stir. It should now start to look like egg fried rice. Please add more egg if you wish.

5 Cook until the cauliflower rice is to your liking and serve. Top with the fresh chives and enjoy.

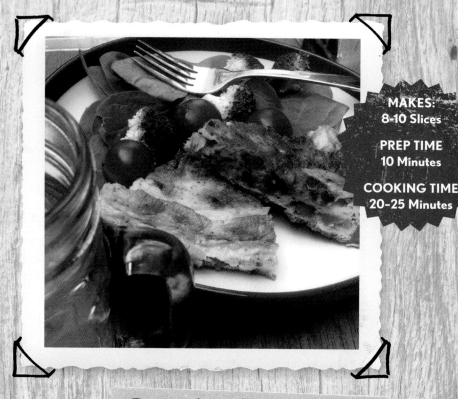

MAKES:
8-10 Slices

PREP TIME
10 Minutes

COOKING TIME
20–25 Minutes

Smoked Salmon
and Squash Frittata

Ingredients

★ 2 tbsp coconut oil
★ 2 cloves garlic, peeled and finely chopped
★ ½ medium butternut squash, peeled and finely chopped
★ 1 onion, peeled and finely chopped
★ 2 tsp smoked paprika
★ ½ tsp cayenne pepper powder
★ 1 pack wild smoked salmon
★ 12 eggs, beaten
★ Celtic Sea or Himalayan Pink salt and freshly ground black pepper

1 Heat the coconut oil in a pan over a medium heat. Add the garlic and cook for one minute before adding the squash and onion. Stir fry for another 4 minutes before adding the paprika, cayenne, salt and pepper and stirring through again.

2 Preheat the broiler.

3 Cook the ingredients for around 10 minutes or until fully cooked before adding the smoked salmon and cooking for a couple of minutes.

4 Add the beaten eggs to the pan and stir slightly. Cook for about 5 minutes until the bottom half has cooked.

5 Now place the pan under the broiler and cook until the frittata is cooked right through.

Marinated Garlic, Honey and Mustard Salmon

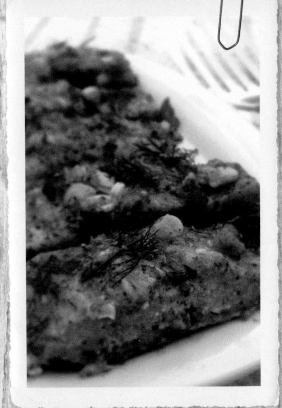

Ingredients

★ 4 fillets of salmon
★ 2 tbsp wholegrain mustard
★ 2 tbsp honey
★ Zest and juice of 1 lemon
★ 3 tbsp olive oil
★ 3 scallions, chopped
★ 2 cloves of garlic, crushed or
   finely chopped
★ 1 red or green chili, deseeded
   and sliced
★ 1 handful fresh dill, chopped
★ Celtic Sea or Himalayan Pink salt
   and freshly ground black pepper

1 Preheat the oven to 350°F.

2 Mix all of the ingredients except the salmon fillets in a large baking dish.

3 Add the salmon fillets and coat each one thoroughly in the marinade.

4 Place in the oven and cook for 15-20 minutes.

5 Once cooked, top with more fresh dill.

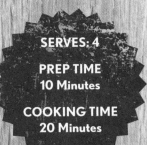

SERVES: 4

PREP TIME
10 Minutes

COOKING TIME
20 Minutes

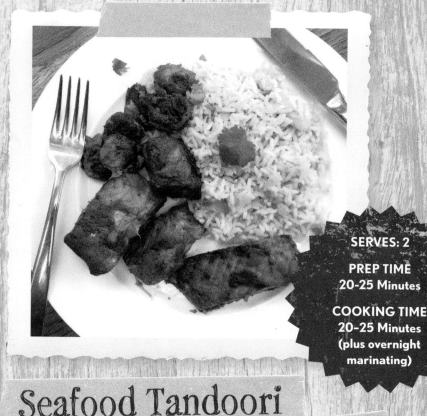

SERVES: 2

PREP TIME
20-25 Minutes

COOKING TIME
20-25 Minutes
(plus overnight
marinating)

Seafood Tandoori
Mixed Grill

Ingredients

★ Juice of 1 lemon
★ 2 tsp Celtic Sea or Himalayan Pink salt
★ 2 tsp paprika
★ ¾ cup (200 ml) can full-fat coconut milk
★ 1-inch piece fresh ginger, peeled
★ 4 cloves garlic, peeled
★ 1 handful fresh cilantro
★ 2 tsp ground coriander
★ 2 tsp ground cumin
★ 1 tsp turmeric
★ ¼ tsp pepper
★ ¼ tsp ground cardamom
★ ⅛ tsp ground cloves
★ ¼-1 tsp chili powder
★ ½ pound (250g) cod fillets
★ ½ pound (250g) salmon fillets
★ ½ pound (250g) jumbo shrimp

TO SERVE
★ Fresh cilantro

1 Place all the ingredients, except for the fish and shrimp, into a food processor and blend into a creamy sauce. You can mix them in a bowl, but make sure you chop the garlic, ginger and cilantro finely if doing this manually.

2 Slice the cod and salmon fillets in half and place in a bowl with the shrimp and marinade sauce. Use your hands to coat each piece in the marinade. Leave in the fridge to marinate for a couple of hours at least, but ideally overnight for maximum flavor.

3 Preheat the oven to 350°F.

4 Place the fish into a baking dish or onto skewers before placing in the oven and cooking for 20-25 minutes or until cooked to your liking.

5 Serve topped with more fresh cilantro.

Simple Spanish Omelet

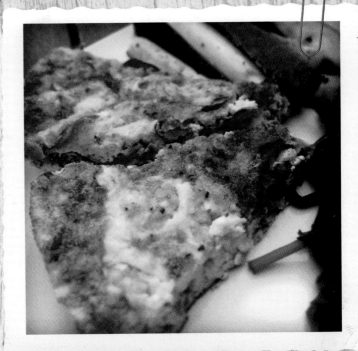

Ingredients

★ 1 tbsp coconut oil
★ 6 eggs, beaten
★ 1 red pepper, thinly sliced
★ 2 cloves garlic, crushed or finely
   chopped
★ 2 ounces (50g) cooked shrimp
★ 2 ounces (50g) wild smoked salmon
★ 3-½ ounces (100g) new potatoes,
   sliced
★ Himalayan Pink or Celtic Sea salt
   and freshly ground black pepper

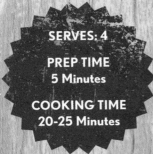

SERVES: 4

PREP TIME
5 Minutes

COOKING TIME
20-25 Minutes

1 Preheat the broiler.

2 Place your new potatoes in a steamer and cook for about 10-12 minutes until soft.

3 As the potatoes cook, heat the coconut oil in a pan over a medium heat.

4 Add the garlic and peppers, and stir well until the peppers soften.

5 Add your new potatoes, salmon and shrimp, and stir fry for one minute.

6 Beat the eggs with seasoning in a bowl, then add to the pan. Stir gently to combine the ingredients, then leave to set and cook for around 4 minutes.

7 After 4 minutes, place the pan under the preheated broiler and continue to cook for another 2-3 minutes or until the top of the tortilla is golden.

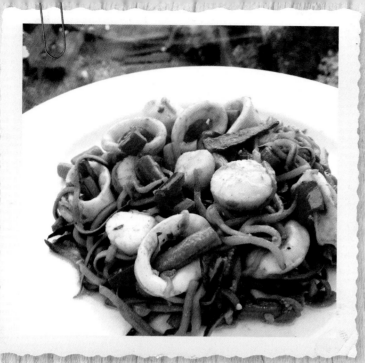

SERVES: 4

PREP TIME
10 Minutes

COOKING TIME
17–20 Minutes

Quick Seafood
Stir Fry

Ingredients

★ 1 tbsp coconut oil
★ 1 red pepper, deseeded and sliced
★ 1 handful string beans, halved
★ 10 cherry tomatoes, halved
★ 2 cloves garlic, peeled and finely chopped
★ 1 heaping tsp smoked paprika
★ ½ tsp chili powder
★ ½ lb (200g) raw scallops
★ ⅔ lb (300g) raw squid rings
★ Celtic Sea or Himalayan Pink salt and freshly ground black pepper
★ 2 large zucchini, julienned

1 Heat the coconut oil in a large frying pan over a medium heat. Add the pepper, string beans, tomatoes and garlic, and stir fry.

2 Stir in the paprika and chili powder, and cook for another 6–8 minutes.

3 Add the scallops and squid rings and coat in the spices. Cook for another 4–5 minutes, stirring occasionally.

4 Finally, add the julienned zucchini, combine all the ingredients and cook for around 3 minutes or until cooked to your liking.

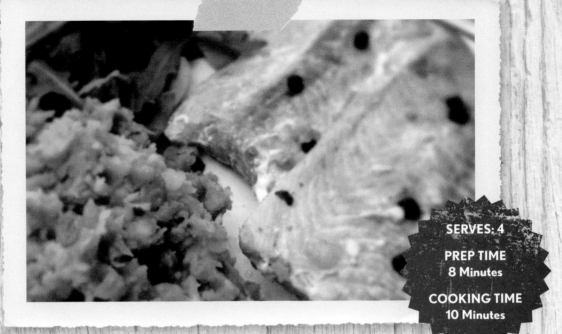

Citrus Salmon With Pea and Avocado Mash

Ingredients

★ 1 tbsp ghee
★ Juice of 1 lemon
★ 2 cloves garlic, finely chopped
★ Himalayan Pink or Celtic Sea salt
  and freshly ground black pepper
  to taste
★ 4 wild salmon fillets

FOR THE MASH:

★ ½ lb (250g) new potatoes, halved
★ ½ lb (250g) frozen peas
★ 1 ripe avocado
★ 1 - 2 tbsp butter
★ Celtic Sea or Himalayan Pink salt
  and freshly ground black pepper

1 Add the new potatoes and peas to a steamer and cook for about 8-10 minutes until soft.

2 While the potatoes are cooking, heat the ghee in a pan over a medium heat and add the garlic, lemon juice, salt and pepper. Cook for about 30 seconds before adding the salmon fillets.

3 Cook the salmon for around about 3-4 minutes on each side.

4 When the potatoes and peas are cooked, drain and place in a bowl. Add the avocado, butter, salt and pepper and mash until smooth.

5 Serve the salmon with the mash and pour over the leftover cooking juices from the salmon.

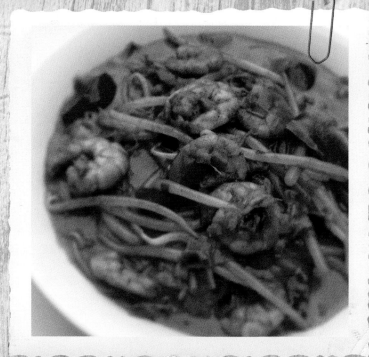

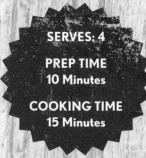

Easy Shrimp Red Thai Curry

Ingredients

★ 1 heaping tbsp coconut oil
★ 2 ½-inch chunk of ginger, peeled and finely chopped
★ 3 cloves garlic, peeled and finely chopped
★ 6 scallions, chopped
★ 3 tsp paprika
★ 1 tsp hot chili powder
★ ½ tsp cinnamon
★ 1 red pepper, chopped
★ 1 red chili, deseeded and finely chopped
★ 2 tbsp tomato purée
★ 2 lemongrass stalks, cut long ways and bashed with a rolling pin
★ Zest of 1 lime
★ 1 lb (500g) jumbo shrimp
★ 2 cups (500 ml) coconut cream
★ 1 tbsp fish sauce
★ Celtic Sea or Himalayan Pink salt and freshly ground black pepper
★ ½ lb (200g) bean sprouts

1 Heat the coconut oil in a large pan, wok or a casserole dish and then add the ginger, garlic, scallions, paprika, chili and cinnamon before stirring and cooking for about 2 minutes, stirring occasionally.

2 Add the pepper, red chili, tomato purée, lemongrass stalks, zest of lime and shrimp, and stir well, coating the shrimp in the tomato purée and spices. Then cook for about 2 minutes, stirring occasionally.

2 Add the coconut cream, fish sauce, salt and pepper and stir well. Simmer for about 3 minutes before adding the bean sprouts and simmering for another 2 minutes.

4 Serve with some white rice or cauliflower rice or just enjoy on its own as we did. We actually wilted some spinach into this at the end, so feel free to give it a try, too, for some added nutrients!

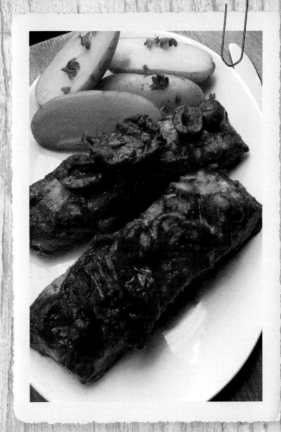

Tomato, Caper and Olive Salmon

Ingredients

★ 2-½ cups (600g) tomato sauce
★ 3 cloves garlic, finely chopped
★ 4 tbsp (80g) capers
★ 10 large green olives, chopped
★ 1 red onion, finely chopped
★ 3 tbsp sun-dried tomatoes in olive oil
★ 6 salmon fillets

1 Preheat the oven to 350°F.

2 Mix all the ingredients except for the salmon in a large baking dish. Add the salmon fillets, ensuring each fillet is nicely topped with the sauce.

3 Place the baking dish into the oven to cook for around 30 minutes.

131

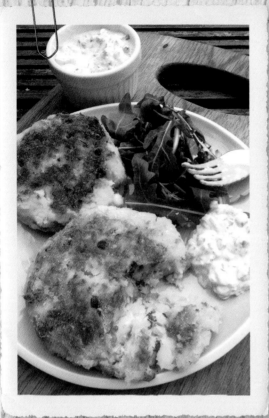

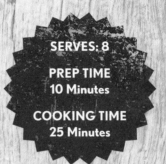

SERVES: 8

PREP TIME
10 Minutes

COOKING TIME
25 Minutes

Fish, Chips
and Mushy Pea Cakes

Ingredients

★ 2-¼ lbs (1 kg) white potatoes, peeled
  and chopped
★ 1-½ lbs (700g) haddock or cod
★ 2 tbsp coconut oil or butter
★ 11 oz (300g) peas
★ 1 handful fresh dill, roughly chopped
★ Celtic Sea or Himalayan Pink salt
  and freshly ground black pepper
★ 3 tbsp rice flour

1 Boil or steam the potatoes for 10-15 minutes until soft.

2 While the potatoes cook, fry the fish fillets in a pan with 1 tablespoon of either coconut oil or butter.

3 When the potatoes are almost cooked, add the peas to the pan to cook for the final few minutes.

4 Place the potatoes and peas in a large bowl with the fresh dill, salt and pepper, and mash the ingredients together.

5 Spread the rice flour out on a plate. Shape the potato mixture into fish cake patties and coat each with a little flour.

6 Heat the remaining coconut oil or butter in a pan over medium heat and cook the fish cakes for around 4 minutes on each side until golden.

7 Serve with salad and homemade tartar sauce (page 227).

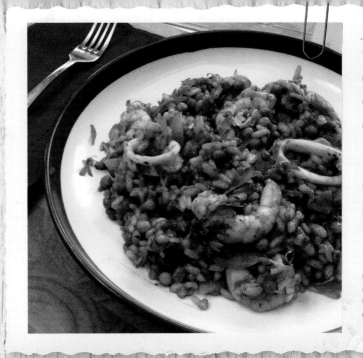

SERVES: 3-4

PREP TIME
10 Minutes

COOKING TIME
25 Minutes

Paella
Pronto

Ingredients

★ 2 tbsp olive oil
★ 1 onion, peeled and chopped
★ 2 cloves garlic, peeled and finely chopped
★ 1 tsp smoked paprika
★ ½ tsp cayenne powder
★ 1 tsp dried thyme
★ 11 oz (300g) paella or risotto rice
★ 14 oz (400g) can chopped tomatoes
★ 1 quart (900 ml) chicken stock
★ Celtic Sea or Himalayan Pink salt and freshly ground black pepper
★ ½ lb (250g) peas
★ ½ lb (250g) raw jumbo shrimp
★ ½ lb (200g) raw squid rings
★ Juice of ½ lemon

TO SERVE
★ 1 handful fresh parsley

1 Heat the olive oil in a large pan over a medium heat before adding the onion and garlic and cooking until soft.

2 Add the smoked paprika, cayenne powder, thyme and rice, and stir well.

3 Add the tomatoes, chicken stock, salt and pepper, and stir well. Simmer for around 15 minutes or until the rice is fully cooked.

4 Add the peas, shrimp and squid rings and stir again. Allow to cook for another 5 minutes or until the shrimp is fully cooked.

5 Squeeze the lemon juice over the top and serve topped with fresh parsley.

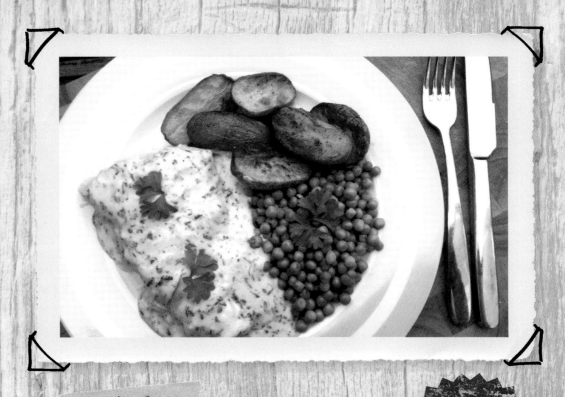

Fish in Parsley Sauce

SERVES: 2

PREP TIME
5 Minutes

COOKING TIME
15 Minutes

Ingredients

★ 2 tbsp coconut oil
★ 2 fillets haddock or cod
★ Celtic Sea or Himalayan Pink salt
  and freshly ground black pepper
★ 1 tbsp of butter
★ 1 tsp onion powder (or use ½ a fresh
  onion, finely chopped)
★ 2 cloves of garlic, peeled and finely
  chopped
★ 1-¾ cup (400 ml) coconut milk
★ 3 oz (80-100g) fresh parsley, finely
  chopped
★ 1 tsp tapioca flour
★ Water

TO SERVE:
★ Peas
★ Roast potatoes, boiled potatoes
  or mash

1 Heat the olive oil in a frying pan over a medium heat and add the fish fillets. Season with salt and pepper and cook for around 5 minutes on each side.

2 As the fish cooks, heat the butter in a pan over a medium heat. Add the garlic and cook for a couple of minutes before adding the coconut milk and onion, then stir well.

3 Bring to a boil, add the parsley and reduce to a simmer for a few minutes.

4 To thicken, mix one teaspoon of tapioca in a cup with a little water and stir into a paste. Add this to the sauce and stir well. If the sauce doesn't thicken enough, repeat this step.

5 Serve the fish and pour over the parsley sauce.

6 Serve with peas and crispy roast potatoes or a creamy mash.

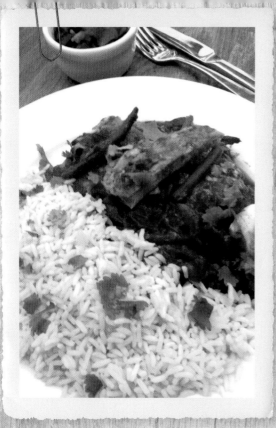

Curried Fish Bake

Ingredients
★ 4 fillets of cod or haddock
★ ½ lb (220g) green beans
★ ½ large onion, finely chopped
★ 3 cloves of garlic, peeled and finely chopped
★ 2 tbsp medium curry powder
★ ½ pint (200 ml) canned coconut milk
★ 14 oz (400g) tomato sauce
★ Celtic Sea or Himalayan Pink salt and freshly ground black pepper

TO SERVE:
★ Rice
★ Wilted spinach

1 Preheat the oven to 350°F.

2 Place the fish fillets in a large casserole dish and scatter over the onions, garlic and green beans.

3 In a separate bowl, mix the tomato sauce, coconut milk and curry powder, and pour over the fish and green beans.

4 Place in the oven to cook for 30-40 minutes.

5 Serve with rice and wilted spinach.

TIP
You can make this just with coconut milk (use 2-½ cups (600 ml) of coconut milk or one 400 ml can and make up with a little stock or bone broth. Alternatively, keep this just a tomato-based sauce and use 2-½ to 3 cups (600-700 ml) of tomato sauce.

Chicken Tandoori Skewers

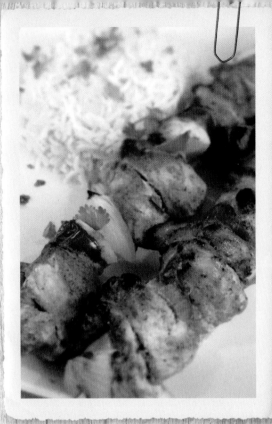

Ingredients

★ 2 pounds (850g) chopped chicken
  (breast, thigh or leg meat)

MARINADE INGREDIENTS

★ Juice of 1 lemon
★ Celtic Sea or Himalayan Pink salt
  and freshly ground black pepper
★ 2 tsp paprika
★ ½ can full fat coconut milk
★ 1 inch piece fresh ginger, peeled
★ 3-4 cloves garlic, crushed
★ 2 tsp ground coriander
★ 2 tsp ground cumin
★ 1 tsp turmeric
★ ¼ tsp pepper
★ ¼ tsp ground cardamom
★ ⅛ tsp ground cloves
★ ¼ -1 tsp chili powder

TO ADD TO SKEWER

★ 1 onion
★ 1 red pepper
★ 1 yellow pepper
★ 1 handful cherry tomatoes

★ Fresh cilantro (optional)

1 Place all the ingredients except the chicken in a bowl and mix well. We used our Nutribullet to blend.

2 Place the chicken in the tandoori marinade and leave for 30 minutes (Note: 2-3 hours or overnight is better to allow the spices to infuse the meat.)

3 After the chicken has been left to marinate, preheat the oven to 350°F.

4 Thread the chicken onto skewers, alternating with slices of onion, pepper and tomato. Place in the oven to cook for 25 minutes and serve topped with fresh cilantro.

SERVES: 4

PREP TIME
10 Minutes

MARINADE TIME
30 Minutes-Overnight

COOKING TIME
25 Minutes

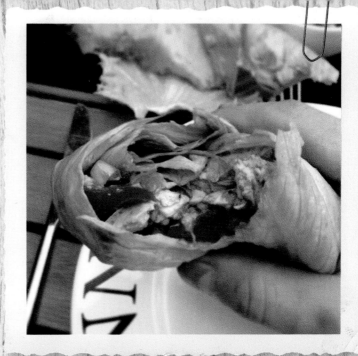

SERVES: 4

PREP TIME
5 Minutes

COOKING TIME
10 Minutes

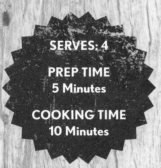

Chicken Fajitas

Ingredients

FOR THE FAJITAS

★ 3 chicken breasts, cut into strips
★ Juice of 2 limes (and a little bit of the pulp too)
★ 2 tbsp dried oregano
★ ½ tsp cayenne pepper powder
★ 1 tsp paprika or smoked paprika
★ ½ tsp cinnamon
★ 1 large onion, chopped
★ 2 bell peppers (red or green), chopped
★ 1 tsp coconut oil
★ 1 large iceberg lettuce, leaves separated
★ Celtic Sea or Himalayan Pink salt and freshly ground black pepper

FOR THE GUACAMOLE

★ 2 avocados
★ Celtic Sea or Himalayan Pink salt

FOR THE SALSA

★ 1 large handful cherry tomatoes
★ 5 scallions, finely chopped
★ 1 small handful fresh cilantro, finely chopped
★ 1 tsp olive oil

1 Place the lime juice, oregano, cayenne pepper, paprika, cinnamon and some salt and pepper in a bowl and mix well. Now add the chicken strips and mix until the chicken is fully covered. (Feel free to leave this to marinate for about 30 minutes to maximize the flavor.)

2 Heat the coconut oil in a pan and add the chicken. Cook for about 2-3 minutes before adding the onions and bell peppers and stirring well. Cook until the chicken is fully cooked and the onions and peppers have softened. While this is cooking through you can prepare the guacamole and salsa.

3 For the guacamole, simply mash the avocados in a bowl with the salt. Easy!

4 For the salsa simply mix the tomatoes, scallions, fresh cilantro and olive oil together in a bowl.

5 Hold the lettuce leaf in your hand, spoon in a portion of the chicken, top with the guacamole and then the salsa. Then fold the leaf around the filling and sink your teeth in.

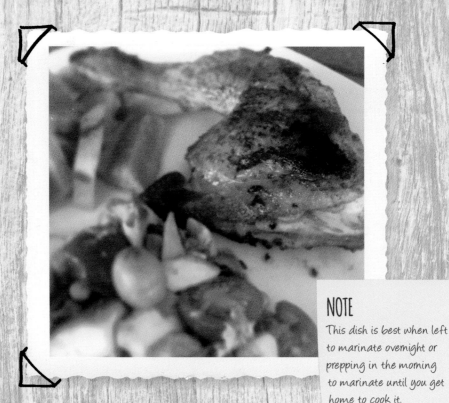

NOTE
This dish is best when left to marinate overnight or prepping in the morning to marinate until you get home to cook it.

Tamari, Ginger and Lime Chicken

Ingredients

★ 3 tbsp tamari
★ 2 cloves garlic, crushed and finely chopped
★ 1-inch cube of ginger, peeled and finely chopped
★ Juice of 1 lime
★ Himalayan Pink or Celtic Sea salt and freshly ground black pepper
★ 1 whole chicken, quartered
★ 2 tbsp coconut oil

SERVES: 4

PREP TIME
5 Minutes

COOKING TIME
35-40 Minutes

1 Add all ingredients except for the coconut oil and chicken into a large bowl and mix together. Then add the chicken and coat thoroughly in the marinade. Leave for the desired time.

2 Preheat the oven to 350°F.

3 Heat the coconut oil in a pan over a medium heat before adding the chicken skin side down and cooking for about 5 minutes or until the skin turns nice and golden.

4 Remove from the pan and place the chicken on a baking dish skin side up and top with any remainder of the marinade. Place in the oven to cook for 35-40 minutes depending on the size of the chicken.

5 Once the chicken is cooked, serve and enjoy.

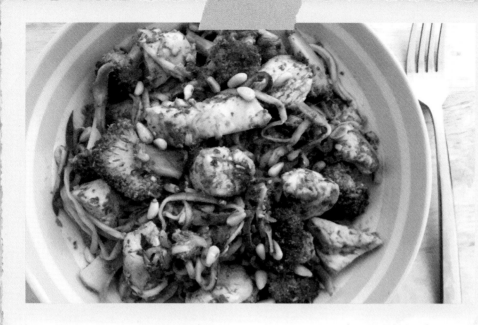

Pesto Chicken with Zucchini

Ingredients

★ 3 skinless chicken breasts, sliced into strips
★ 5 large zucchini, sliced julienne style
★ 2 cloves garlic, crushed
★ 2 tbsp olive oil or butter for cooking
★ 1 pound (400g) broccoli, broken into florets and thinly sliced
★ ¾ cup (180g) green pesto
★ 3 tbsp (40g) toasted pine nuts

SERVES: 4

PREP TIME
8 Minutes

COOKING TIME
10 Minutes

1 Lightly toast the pine nuts in a pan without any oil for 2-3 minutes until golden. Be careful not to let them burn. Remove from the pan and set to one side.

2 Heat the cooking oil in a pan and add the broccoli and chicken. Stir fry for 4-5 minutes.

3 Add the crushed garlic and cook for another 3 minutes.

4 Add the pesto, half the pine nuts and zucchini spaghetti and stir fry thoroughly.

5 Cook until the zucchini softens; be careful not to let it get too soggy.

6 Serve and add the remaining pine nuts on top.

SERVES: 4

PREP TIME
5 Minutes
(Although we
recommend overnight)

COOKING TIME
35-40 Minutes

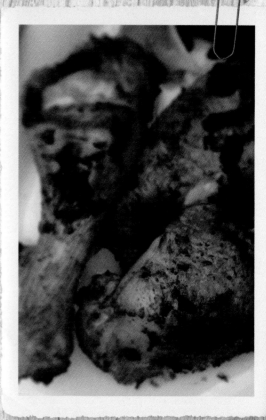

Pimped Up Peri Peri Chicken

Ingredients

★ 4 chicken thighs (skin on, bone in)
★ 4 chicken drumsticks
★ 1 heaping tsp ground ginger
★ 1 heaping tsp ground smoked paprika
★ 1 level tsp cayenne pepper powder
  (more if you want more kick)
★ 1 heaping tsp dried oregano
★ 2 cloves garlic, crushed or
  finely chopped
★ Himalayan Pink or Celtic Sea salt and
  freshly ground black pepper
★ 2 tbsp olive oil/macadamia oil
★ 3 tbsp tomato purée
★ Juice and zest of 1 lemon

1 Preheat the oven to 400°F.

2 Place the ginger, paprika, cayenne, oregano, garlic, salt and pepper in a large bowl and mix well. Add the oil, tomato purée, lemon juice/zest and mix together to form a paste.

3 Now add the chicken and using your hands coat the chicken in the marinade. If you can, marinate the chicken overnight.

4 Place the chicken on a baking pan and put in the top half of the oven. Cook on the higher heat for 10 minutes before turning the heat down to 350°F.

5 Cook for another 25-30 minutes or until fully cooked.

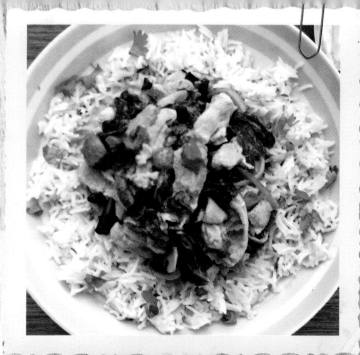

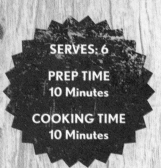
Ingredients

FOR THE PASTE

★ 3 lemongrass stalks, outer layer removed and finely sliced

★ 6 medium hot green chilies, deseeded and finely chopped

★ 2 cloves garlic, peeled and finely chopped

★ 2 inch piece of fresh ginger, peeled and grated

★ 2 shallots, peeled and finely chopped

★ 1 large handful fresh cilantro, roughly chopped

★ 1 tbsp coriander seeds, crushed

★ 1 tsp cumin powder

★ Zest of 2 limes

★ Juice of 1 lime

★ 1 tbsp fish sauce

★ 3 tbsp olive oil

★ Freshly ground black pepper to taste

FOR THE SAUCE

★ 1 tbsp coconut oil

★ 1 clove garlic, peeled and finely chopped

★ ½ pound (250)g cremini/baby portobello mushrooms

★ 2 lbs of chicken thigh, deboned and cut into strips

★ 1-¾ cup (400ml) coconut milk

★ 1 small handful fresh basil, roughly chopped

★ 1 large handful spinach

TO SERVE

★ Steamed greens and mango sticky rice (see page 189)

SAY THAT QUICKLY 5 TIMES! ☺

Thigh Thai Green Curry

1 Place all the paste ingredients into a food processor and blend into a paste.

2 Heat the coconut oil in a large pan or saucepan. Add the garlic and allow to cook for around one minute, being careful not to burn.

3 Add the chicken strips and mushrooms and pan fry until golden. Add the curry paste mixture and stir well.

4 Add the coconut milk and fresh basil and stir again.

5 Bring to a boil, then reduce the heat to a simmer and cook for 8 minutes. Stir occasionally.

6 Remove from the heat and stir in the spinach. Allow to wilt down and serve.

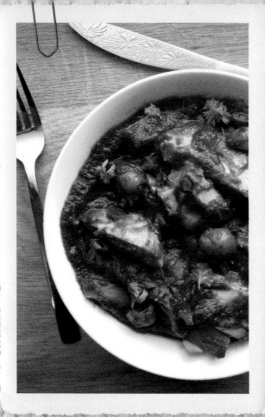

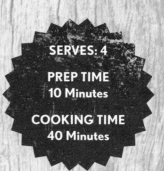

SERVES: 4

PREP TIME
10 Minutes

COOKING TIME
40 Minutes

Spanish Style Chicken

Ingredients

★ 1 tbsp olive oil
★ 4 cloves garlic, peeled and chopped
★ 1 small white onion, peeled and chopped
★ 1 leek, sliced
★ 4 chicken breasts, chopped
★ 2 tsp paprika
★ 1 tsp oregano
★ 1 tsp thyme
★ ½-1 tsp Himalayan Pink or Celtic Sea salt
★ ½ tsp black pepper
★ 1 handful olives, halved
★ 2-¾ cups (680g) tomato purée
★ ¾ cup (200 ml) chicken stock
★ 4 sweet or white potatoes, peeled and sliced

1 Heat the olive oil in a large saucepan over medium heat and add the garlic, onions, leeks and stir well. Sauté for 3-4 minutes until the onions and leeks start to soften.

2 Add the chicken and sauté for another 2-3 minutes until the chicken starts to brown. Add the paprika, thyme, oregano, salt and pepper, and stir well, coating all the ingredients in the spices.

3 Add the olives, tomato sauce, chicken stock and potatoes. Bring to a simmer and cook for 30 minutes.

4 Season further if required and serve either on its own or with steamed greens.

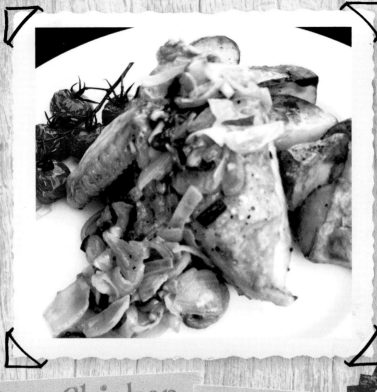

Crispy Chicken in a Tarragon Sauce

SERVES: 2

PREP TIME
5 Minutes

COOKING TIME
40-50 Minutes

Ingredients

★ 2 large chicken breasts (bone in)
★ 2 tbsp olive oil
★ 2 cloves garlic, peeled and finely chopped
★ 1 onion, chopped
★ 6 ounces (150g) mushrooms, sliced
★ ½ cup (120ml) coconut milk
★ 1 cup (240ml) chicken stock
★ 1 handful fresh tarragon, roughly chopped
★ Celtic Sea or Himalayan Pink salt and freshly ground black pepper

1 Preheat the oven to 350°F.

2 Place the chicken breasts on a baking tray and put in the oven to cook for 40-50 minutes or until fully cooked.

3 Just before the chicken is fully cooked, heat the olive oil in a pan over a medium heat. Add the garlic, onion and mushrooms. Stir and cook for a few minutes.

4 Add the coconut milk and chicken stock, and stir.

5 Add the fresh tarragon, salt and pepper, and bring the sauce to a boil. Turn down the heat and simmer for another 5 minutes or until the sauce has reached the thickness you desire.

6 Remove the chicken from the oven and serve topped with the sauce.

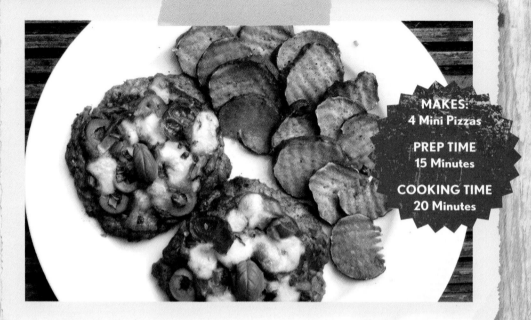

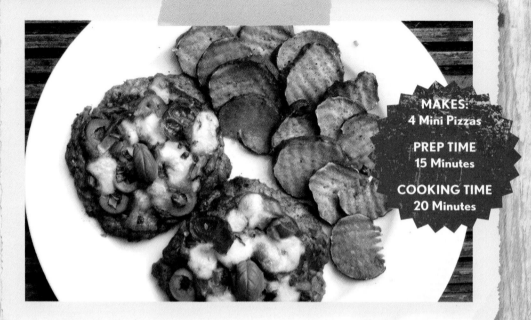

MAKES:
4 Mini Pizzas

PREP TIME
15 Minutes

COOKING TIME
20 Minutes

Mini Protein Pizzas

Ingredients

FOR THE PIZZA BASE

★ 1 pound (500g) ground chicken
★ 1 heaping tbsp tomato purée
★ 1 clove garlic, peeled and finely chopped
★ 1 tsp mixed herbs
★ 1 tsp smoked paprika
★ Celtic Sea or Himalayan Pink salt and freshly ground black pepper

FOR THE SAUCE AND TOPPING

★ 5 tbsp tomato sauce
★ 1 tsp oregano
★ Celtic Sea or Himalayan Pink salt and freshly ground black pepper
★ 4 olives, finely sliced
★ ½ green pepper, deseeded and finely chopped
★ 4 cherry tomatoes, finely sliced
★ Half a mozzarella ball, chopped
★ Fresh basil, roughly chopped

1 Preheat the oven to 350°F.

2 Add the chicken, tomato purée, garlic, mixed herbs, smoked paprika, salt and pepper in a large bowl, and mix together thoroughly with your hands.

3 Use a little olive oil or butter to grease a baking tray.

4 Shape the chicken mixture into four pizza bases. Be careful not to make the bases too thick – around ½-inch is ideal—and place on the baking tray.

5 Make the pizza sauce by mixing the tomato sauce and oregano in a bowl with some seasoning.

6 Top each pizza base with the sauce, leaving a little space at the edge of each base.

7 Top each pizza with olives, cherry tomatoes, mozzarella and fresh basil before placing in the oven to cook for 20 minutes.

SERVES: 3-4

PREP TIME
10 Minutes (overnight
marinating is best)

COOKING TIME
12-15 Minutes

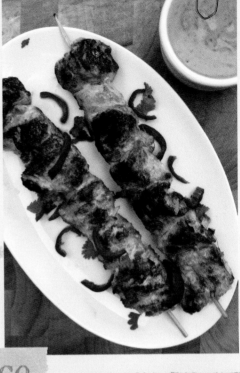

Chicken Skewers with Almond Satay Sauce

Ingredients

FOR THE CHICKEN

★ 4 chicken breasts, diced
★ 1 small chunk of ginger, peeled and finely chopped
★ 2 cloves garlic, peeled and finely chopped
★ Zest and juice of 1 lime
★ 1 tbsp tamari
★ 1 tbsp medium curry powder
★ 1 tsp honey
★ 1 tbsp coconut oil

FOR THE SATAY SAUCE

★ 6 ounces (160g) almond butter
★ ½ cup (120ml) coconut milk
★ ¼ cup (50-60ml) water if needed
★ 2 tbsp honey
★ ½-1 tsp cayenne pepper powder
★ Himalayan Pink or Celtic Sea salt to taste

1 Place all the ingredients for the chicken except the coconut oil into a bowl. Using your hands coat the chicken pieces in the marinade. Ideally leave overnight, but if short on time you can cook immediately or marinate for 30-60 minutes.

2 Place the chicken pieces onto wooden skewers.

3 Heat the coconut oil in a frying pan over a medium heat and add the chicken skewers.

4 Cook for around 12-15 minutes, turning occasionally to cook through.

5 While the skewers cook, prepare the satay sauce. Place all the ingredients in a saucepan (add the water gradually so it doesn't become too runny too quickly— you can always add a little more if needed). Warm over a medium heat and stir. Keep cooking, stirring occasionally, until the sauce is heated through and reaches the desired consistency.

6 Serve with rice and stir-fried vegetables.

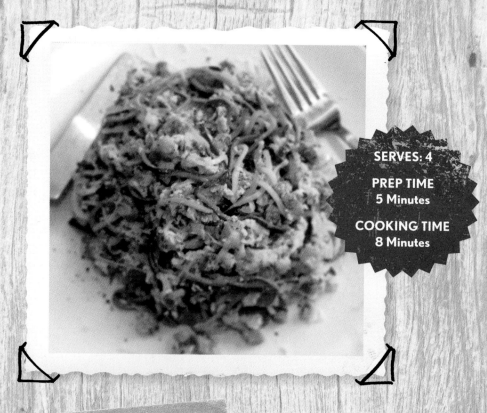

Zucchini Carbonara

Ingredients

★ 4 medium zucchini (peeled with a julienne peeler)
★ 7 ounces (200g) pancetta, chopped or cubed
★ 2 tbsp olive oil
★ 3 cloves garlic, crushed
★ 1 large handful fresh parsley, finely chopped
★ 3 eggs, beaten
★ 4 Tbsp (60g) Parmesan cheese, grated
★ Black pepper
★ Olive oil for cooking

TIP

Don't cook the zucchini for too long as they quickly go soggy. Adapt this dish by adding shrimp, smoked salmon or chicken.

1 Heat the olive oil in a pan over a medium heat. While this heats, slice your zucchini with a julienne peeler.

2 Once the pan has heated, add the pancetta and stir fry until lightly browned.

3 Add the crushed garlic and fresh parsley and cook for a few seconds before adding the zucchini spaghetti and stir frying for another 3–4 minutes.

4 Add the beaten eggs and half of the grated cheese and mix all of the ingredients together.

5 Once the eggs and zucchini have cooked and achieved a creamy texture, remove from the heat.

6 Top with black pepper, the remaining Parmesan cheese and some fresh parsley.

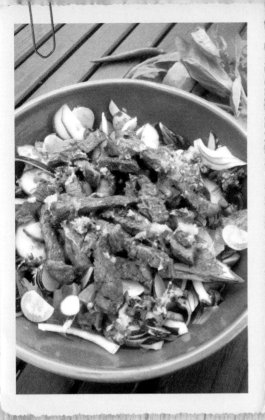

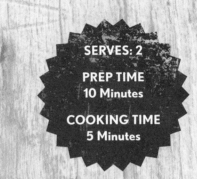

SERVES: 2

PREP TIME
10 Minutes

COOKING TIME
5 Minutes

Thai Style Steak Salad

Ingredients
★ 2 7-ounce (200g) rump steaks

TO MAKE THE DRESSING
★ Zest and juice of 3 limes
★ 2 tbsp tamari
★ Freshly ground black pepper
★ 1 dice-sized piece of ginger, peeled and grated
★ 1 green or red chili
★ 1 tsp xylitol
★ 1 handful fresh cilantro, finely chopped
★ 1 tbsp coconut oil

FOR THE SALAD
★ 7 ounces (200g) cherry tomatoes, quartered
★ ½ cucumber, sliced
★ 7 ounces (200g) radishes, sliced
★ 1 red onion, sliced
★ 1 handful fresh mint, roughly broken
★ 1 handful fresh basil, roughly broken

1 Mix the tamari, zest and juice of one lime and pepper in a bowl.

2 Slice the steaks into strips and add them to the bowl, then coat fully in the mixture.

3 Mix the remaining lime zest/lime juice with the ginger, chili, xylitol and cilantro to make the dressing.

4 Heat the coconut oil in a pan over a medium heat before adding the marinated steak strips. Stir fry for 3-4 minutes or to your liking. Leave to cool while you mix the salad ingredients together.

5 Place the steak strips on top of the salad and drizzle the dressing over the top.

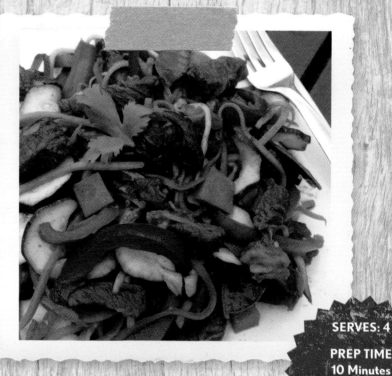

SERVES: 4

PREP TIME
10 Minutes

COOKING TIME
12 Minutes

Beef 5 A Day Stir Fry

Ingredients

★ 2 tbsp coconut oil
★ 2 cloves garlic, finely chopped
★ 1-inch piece of ginger, peeled and finely chopped
★ ½-1 red chili
★ 1 pound (500g) sirloin steak, cut into strips
★ 1 red pepper
★ 1 green pepper
★ 3-½ ounces (100g) snow peas
★ 2 carrots, julienned (keep the middles and chop thinly to go into the stir fry)
★ 3 zucchini, julienned (keep the middles and chop thinly to go into the stir fry)
★ 3 tbsp tomato purée
★ 3 tbsp honey/xylitol
★ 2 tbsp tamari

1 Heat the coconut oil in a large pan or wok over a medium heat, then add the garlic, ginger and chili, and stir fry before adding the steak strips. Cook for 3 minutes, stirring occasionally.

2 Add the peppers, snow peas and the middle of the carrots/zucchini (sliced), and stir fry for 4 minutes or until the vegetables start to soften.

3 Mix the tomato purée, honey and tamari together in a bowl and pour over the meat and vegetables. Stir fry a little before adding the julienned zucchini and carrots.

4 Mix all the ingredients together and cook until the carrots have softened slightly.

MAKES:
8 Scotch Eggs

PREP TIME
10-15 Minutes

COOKING TIME
25-30 Minutes

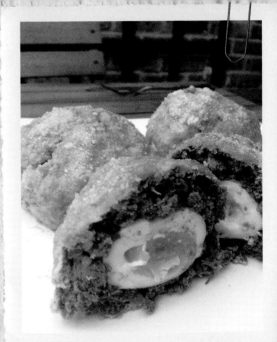

Mexican Style Lamb Scotch Eggs

Ingredients

★ 10 eggs (2 for the coating)
★ 1-¾ pounds (800g) ground lamb
★ 1 green pepper, finely chopped
★ 1 handful jalepenos, finely chopped
   (well-drained and dabbed with
   kitchen towel to get rid of excess
   moisture)
★ 1 large handful fresh cilantro,
   roughly chopped
★ 3 heaping tsp tomato purée
★ 3 tsp paprika
★ 2 tsp dried oregano
★ 1 tsp cayenne pepper powder
★ 1 tsp garlic flakes or 2 fresh cloves
   garlic, finely chopped
★ A good pinch of Celtic Sea or
   Himalayan Pink salt
★ 6 Tbsp. (100g) ground almonds

TIP

Handle the eggs with care when molding the meat around them, as you don't want them to break.

1 Preheat the oven to 350°F. Mix the lamb, green pepper, jalepenos, cilantro, tomato purée, paprika, oregano, cayenne, garlic and salt in a large bowl and mix well using your hands. Be sure to thoroughly combine all the ingredients. Keep two eggs to one side for the coating but soft boil the others.

2 Bring some water to a boil in a saucepan, add your eggs and then bring to a boil again for 4 minutes. After 4 minutes, immediately add them to a bowl of cold water so they stop them cooking even more (this is an attempt to keep a slightly runny or at least soft yolk). Make sure you start the 4 minutes once the eggs are boiling and not before or they won't cook long enough.

3 Spread your ground almonds out on a plate and beat the other two eggs in a bowl. You are now ready to make the Scotch eggs.

4 Remove the shells from your eggs. Shape the meat around the egg. Keep molding it and pushing the gaps together with your fingers. Splash your fingers in some cold water while molding the meat around the eggs. This makes it a lot easier to shape. Repeat until all of the eggs are covered. The meat layer should be roughly ⅜-inch thick. If it's too thin, the meat will split when in the oven.

5 Then one-by-one roll the eggs in the beaten egg then in the ground almonds to coat them completely. Place them in an oven dish, ideally on some sort of baking pan so the juices can drip from the Scotch eggs. Place in the oven and cook for 25 minutes or until thoroughly cooked.

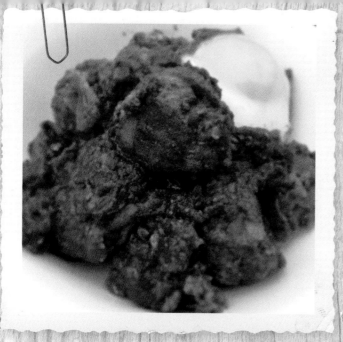

Moroccan Style Meatballs Topped with Eggs

Ingredients

★ 1 pound (500g) of ground beef
★ 2 onions, peeled and chopped
★ 1 tbsp olive oil
★ 4 tsp Ras el Hanout spice mix
★ 14 ounces (400g) chopped tomatoes
★ 3 cloves garlic, crushed
★ 4 eggs
★ Celtic Sea or Himalayan Pink salt and freshly ground black pepper

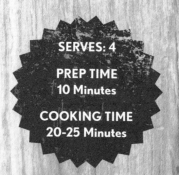

SERVES: 4

PREP TIME
10 Minutes

COOKING TIME
20-25 Minutes

TO MAKE THE MEATBALLS

1 Mix the ground beef, onion, two teaspoons of Ras el Hanout and one egg in a bowl. Season with Himalayan Pink salt and pepper. Mix thoroughly using your hands.

2 Make the mixture into meatballs about the size of a golf ball. It should make around 12.

3 Heat the olive oil in a pan, then add the meatballs. Cook for about 4-5 minutes until they start to brown nicely.

TO MAKE THE SAUCE

1 Add the other onion and crushed garlic, and cook until onion starts to soften.

2 Now add the chopped tomatoes and remaining Ras el Hanout spice mix and season with Himalayan Pink salt and pepper. Stir to coat the meatballs in the sauce.

3 Allow this to simmer for about 10-12 minutes.

4 Create three gaps in the mixture and crack an egg into each. Loosely cover the pan with foil or a lid and simmer for another 4-5 minutes until the egg whites are cooked.

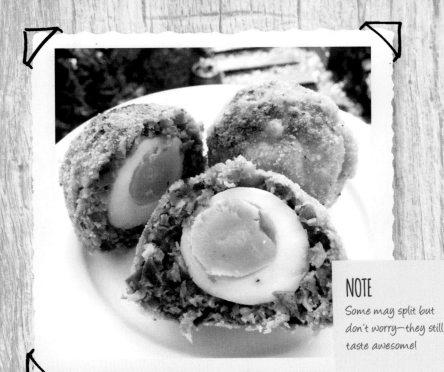

NOTE
Some may split but don't worry—they still taste awesome!

Italian Style Scotch Eggs

Ingredients

★ 12 eggs (2 for coating)
★ 12 gluten-free sausages
★ 2 large handfuls sun-dried tomatoes in olive oil, roughly chopped
★ 1 handful green olives, chopped
★ 6 tbsp (100g) ground almonds

MAKES:
10 Scotch Eggs

PREP TIME
10–15 Minutes

COOKING TIME
25–30 Minutes

1 Bring a large saucepan of water to a boil, add 10 of the eggs and bring back to a boil. Cook for 4 minutes. As soon as the time is up, pour the hot water out and replace with cold water to stop the eggs cooking further.

2 Preheat the oven to 350°F.

3 Remove the skins from your sausages and place the meat in a large bowl with the tomatoes and olives. Use your hands to mix the ingredients together thoroughly.

4 Peel the boiled eggs and spread the ground almonds out on a plate. Place the two remaining eggs in a bowl and beat.

5 Carefully wrap the meat mixture around each egg until the egg is completely covered. Have a bowl of water nearby and wet your hands a little to prevent the mixture from sticking to your hands when shaping the meat around the egg.

6 Once each egg is covered, dip in the beaten egg and roll in the ground almonds, then place on a baking tray and into the oven for 25-30 minutes.

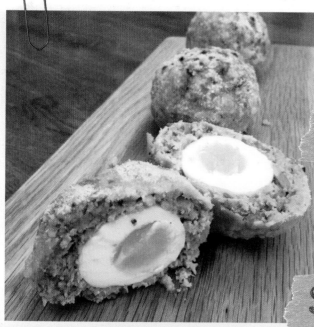

Pork, Apple and Fennel Scotch Eggs

Ingredients

★ 12 eggs (2 for the coating)
★ 1 tbsp of butter
★ 1 large tart apple, chopped into small chunks
★ 1 tbsp xylitol
★ 12 gluten-free sausages
★ 2-3 tsp fennel seeds
★ 6 Tbsp (100g) ground almonds
★ Celtic Sea or Himalayan Pink salt and freshly ground black pepper

MAKES:
10 Scotch Eggs

PREP TIME
15 Minutes

COOKING TIME
25–35 Minutes

1 Preheat the oven to 350°F.

2 Bring a pan of water to a boil and add 10 of the eggs. Bring to a boil again and cook for 4 minutes before immediately placing the eggs into cold water to stop them from cooking further.

3 Heat the butter in a pan over a medium heat and add the apple chunks to cook for about 5 minutes, stirring occasionally. Add the xylitol and cook for another few minutes until softened.

4 Remove the skins from the sausages and place the meat in a large bowl. Then add the cooked apple and fennel and mix all the ingredients together thoroughly with your hands.

5 Beat the two remaining eggs in a bowl. Spread the ground almonds on a plate and add a little salt and pepper.

6 Shape a handful of the sausage mixture around each egg. Aim for a layer about ⅓-inch thick. Have a bowl of water handy, as wetting your hands a little to apply the meat prevents it from sticking to your hands.

7 Coat each Scotch egg in the beaten egg and roll in the ground almonds.

8 Place each Scotch egg on a baking tray and put in the oven to cook for 25 minutes.

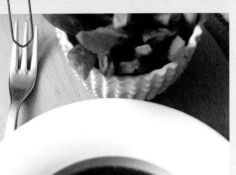

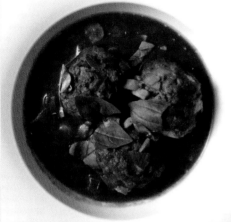

Smoky
Pork Meatballs

Ingredients

FOR THE MEATBALLS

★ 2 pounds (1 kg) ground pork
★ 3 tsp smoked paprika
★ 1 tsp cayenne pepper powder
★ 2-3 tbsp tomato purée
★ 1 onion, peeled and finely chopped
★ 2 large carrots, grated
★ Celtic Sea or Himalayan Pink salt
   and freshly ground black pepper

FOR THE SAUCE

★ 2 24-ounce (2 700g) jars
   tomato purée
★ 7 ounces (200g) mushrooms, halved
   and sliced
★ 6 ounces (180g) cherry tomatoes,
   quartered
★ 2 heaping tsp dried oregano
★ Celtic Sea or Himalayan Pink salt
   and freshly ground black pepper

TO SERVE

★ Fresh basil
★ Sweet potato chips

1 Preheat the oven to 350°F.

2 Mix all the meatball ingredients together in a large bowl thoroughly using your hands and shape into meatballs around the size of a golf ball.

3 For the sauce, use a large baking dish (or two smaller ones) and place all the sauce ingredients in the baking dish. Mix well.

4 Add your meatballs to the sauce, but don't cover the tops of the meatballs with the sauce.

5 Place in the oven to cook for 30 minutes or until fully cooked.

6 Top with some fresh basil and enjoy with some sweet potato chips.

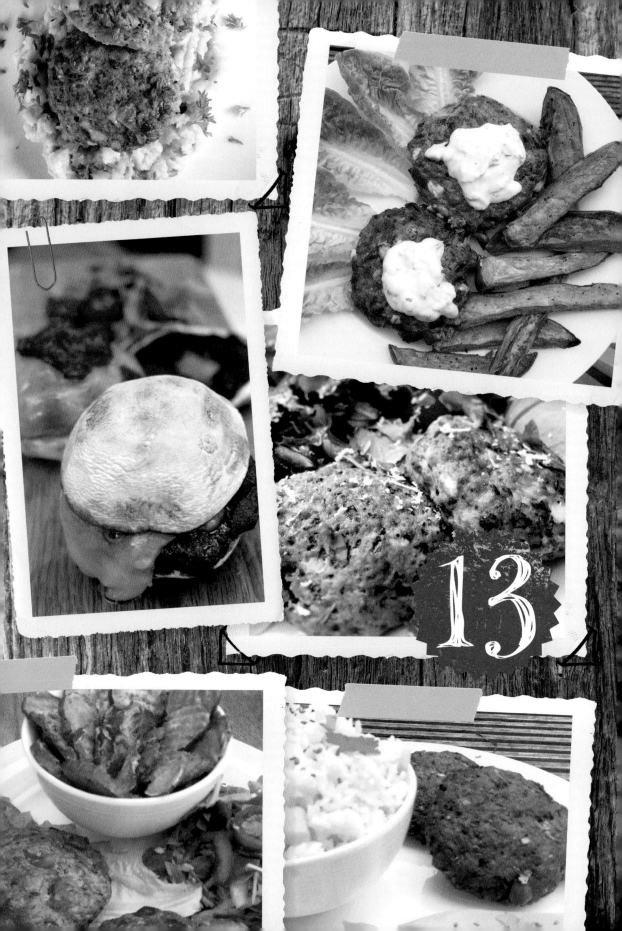

13

BURGER SHACK

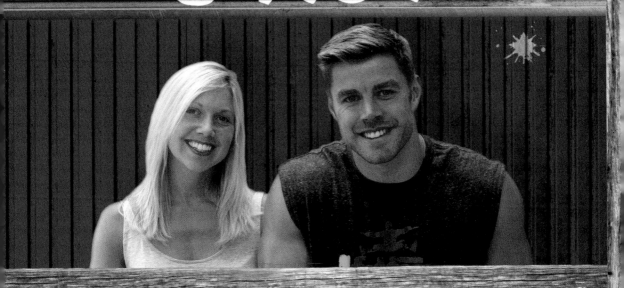

MENU

Pork, Apple & Leek Burgers

Smokey Salmon Burger

Greek Salad Burgers

Curry in a Burger

Basic Beefy & Cheesy Burger

Turkey, Chorizo & Red Pepper Burger

Pesto Turkey Burgers

Greek Style Lamb Burger

Lamb, Pea and Mint Burgers

Oriental Pork Burgers

Pork, Apple and Leek Burgers

Ingredients

* 1 pound (500g) ground pork
* 1 medium tart apple, chopped
* 1 small leek, finely chopped
* 1 garlic clove, finely chopped
* 1 tbsp coconut oil or butter
* 2 tsp dried thyme
* Himalayan Pink or Celtic Sea salt and freshly ground black pepper

1 Preheat the oven to 350°F.

2 Place the ground pork in a mixing bowl.

3 Heat your oil or butter in a pan over a medium heat and add the apple, leek and garlic. Cook for around 5 minutes, stirring occasionally until everything starts to soften.

4 Add the cooked mixture to the pork in the mixing bowl with the thyme, salt and pepper. Using clean hands, mix all the ingredients together before dividing into 5-6 burger patties and placing them on a baking pan or oven dish.

5 Place in the oven to cook for 20-25 minutes or until cooked.

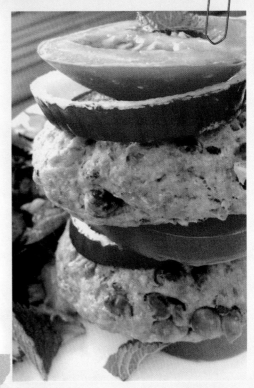

Lamb, Pea and Mint Burgers

Ingredients

* 1 pound (500g) ground lamb
* 7 ounces (200g) peas
* 1 handful fresh mint, finely chopped
* 1 clove garlic, finely chopped
* 1 heaping tsp mustard powder
* 2 tbsp apple cider vinegar
* Himalayan Pink or Celtic Sea salt and freshly ground black pepper

1 Preheat the oven to 350°F.

2 Place your peas in a saucepan, cover with water and bring to a boil. Simmer for 5 minutes or until soft. Drain and mash slightly.

3 Mix all the ingredients together in a large bowl. Using your hands, make 4 burger patties and place on a baking tray

4 Cook in the oven for 20 minutes or until cooked to your liking.

MAKES:
4 Large Burgers

PREP TIME
5 Minutes

COOKING TIME
20-25 Minutes

MAKES:
6 Burgers

PREP TIME
10 Minutes

COOKING TIME
25 Minutes

Quick Homemade Tzatziki

★ 11 ounces (300g) yogurt
★ 1 cucumber, grated and drained
★ 2 cloves garlic, minced
★ 2 tbsp fresh lemon juice
★ 2 tbsp fresh dill, chopped
★ 2 tbsp fresh mint, finely chopped
★ Celtic Sea or Himalayan Pink salt
  and black pepper to taste

In a bowl mix together the yogurt, cucumber, garlic, lemon juice and dill. Season and chill before serving.

SERVES: 6-8
PREP TIME: 10 Minut es

Greek Salad Burgers

Ingredients

* 1 pound (500g) ground chicken or turkey
* 1 handful cherry tomatoes, finely chopped
* 1 small red onion, finely chopped
* 1 handful green or black olives, finely chopped
* 4 ounces (120g) feta cheese, chopped or crumbled
* 1 heaping tbsp tomato purée
* 1-2 tbsp olive oil
* 2 tsp mixed herbs
* Celtic Sea or Himalayan Pink salt and freshly ground black pepper

1 Preheat the oven to 350°F.

2 Place all the ingredients together in a large bowl and combine thoroughly with your hands.

3 Shape into 6 patties and place on a baking pan or oven dish in the oven to cook for 20-25 minutes.

4 Serve with sweet potato wedges, homemade tzatziki and a romaine lettuce wrap.

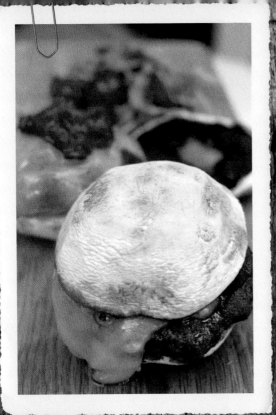

MAKES:
4 Burgers

PREP TIME
10 Minutes

COOKING TIME
20-25 Minutes

The Basic
Beefy and Cheesy
Burger

Ingredients

* 1 pound (500g) ground beef
* 1/2 tsp cayenne pepper powder
* 1 tsp smoked paprika
* 1 tsp garlic powder
* 1 tsp onion powder
* 1 tbsp tomato purée
* Celtic Sea or Himalayan Pink salt and freshly ground black pepper
* A few slices of cheddar cheese to top the burgers

TO SERVE
* Portobello mushroom buns (optional)

1 Preheat the oven to 350°F.

2 Mix all the ingredients thoroughly in a large bowl with your hands.

3 Shape into 4 patties and place on a baking pan or baking tray in the oven for 20-25 minutes.

4 Once cooked, remove the burgers from the oven and top with some cheddar cheese slices. Return to the oven to melt the cheese a little.

5 Serve with the Homemade BBQ Sauce on page 229 in a portobello mushroom bun.

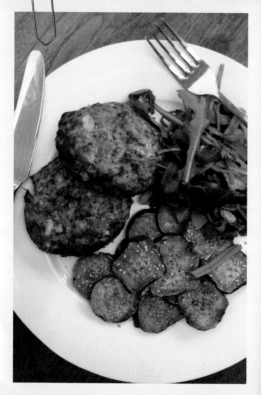

Oriental Pork Burgers

Ingredients
* 1-2/3 pound (750g) ground pork
* 2 dice-sized cubes of ginger, peeled and finely chopped
* 2 cloves garlic, peeled and finely chopped
* 5 scallions, thinly sliced
* 1 tbsp toasted sesame seed oil
* 1 tbsp tamari
* Celtic Sea or Himalayan Pink salt and freshly ground black pepper

1 Preheat the oven to 350°F.

2 Place all the ingredients together in a large bowl and combine thoroughly with your hands. Shape into 6 patties.

3 Place on a baking tray in the oven for 20-25 minutes or until cooked to your liking.

MAKES:
6 Burgers

PREP TIME
6 Minutes

COOKING TIME
20-25 Minutes

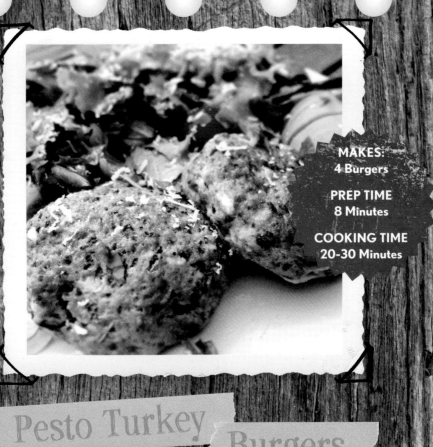

MAKES:
4 Burgers

PREP TIME
8 Minutes

COOKING TIME
20-30 Minutes

Pesto Turkey Burgers

Ingredients
* 1 large handful fresh basil
* 1 ripe avocado peeled, halved and stone removed
* 2 cloves garlic, crushed
* 4 Tbsp (60g) toasted pine nuts
* Juice of 1 lemon
* 2 tbsp olive oil
* Celtic Sea or Himalayan Pink salt and freshly ground black pepper
* 4 Tbsp (60g) grated Parmesan, leaving a little to serve
* 1 pound (400g) ground turkey

1 Preheat the oven to 350°F.

2 Prepare your pesto by placing the basil, garlic, avocado, olive oil, lemon juice, nuts, salt and pepper in a blender and mix for around 20-30 seconds. Feel free to add a little water if you prefer a thinner consistency. Taste and add more basil or seasoning if you wish.

3 In a mixing bowl, combine the pesto, grated Parmesan and ground turkey.

4 Shape into 4 large burger patties and place on a baking tray. Cook for 20-30 minutes, depending on your oven. Be sure to check they are fully cooked.

5 Have these with some sweet potato fries or in a lettuce wrap. Top the burgers with a little more grated Parmesan if you wish and enjoy!

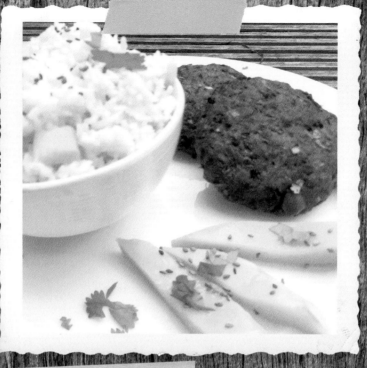

Curry in a Burger

Ingredients

* 1-2/3 pound (750g) ground beef
* 1 jalepeno pepper, seeded and finely chopped (you can use canned)
* 1 small handful fresh mint, chopped
* 1 small handful fresh cilantro, chopped
* 2 cloves garlic, peeled and finely chopped
* 1 dice-size cube of fresh ginger, peeled and grated
* 2 tsp curry powder
* Celtic Sea or Himalayan Pink salt and freshly ground black pepper

1 Preheat the oven to 350°F.

2 Place all the ingredients together in a large bowl and combine thoroughly with your hands. Shape into 6 patties.

3 Place on a baking dish or baking tray in the oven for 20-25 minutes or until cooked to your liking.

MAKES:
6 Burgers

PREP TIME
5 Minutes

COOKING TIME
20-25 Minutes

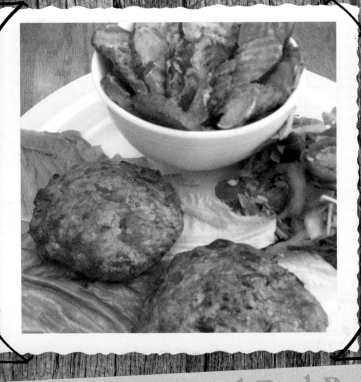

Turkey, Chorizo and Red Pepper Burgers

Ingredients
* 1-2/3 pound (750g) ground turkey
* 7 ounces (200g) chorizo, chopped into small pieces
* 1 red pepper, deseeded and chopped into small pieces
* 1 handful fresh parsley, finely chopped
* 1 tbsp tomato purée

1 Preheat the oven to 350°F.

2 Place all the ingredients together in a large bowl and combine thoroughly with your hands. Shape into 6 patties.

3 Place on a baking dish or baking tray in the oven for 20-25 minutes or until cooked to your liking.

MAKES:
6 Burgers

PREP TIME
5 Minutes

COOKING TIME
20-25 Minutes

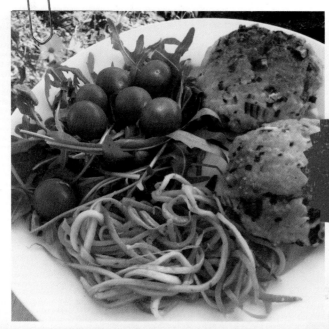

MAKES:
4-6 Burgers

PREP TIME
10 Minutes

COOKING TIME
8-10 Minutes

Smoky Salmon Burgers

Ingredients
* 1 pound (500g) skinless salmon fillets
* 4 ounces (120g) smoked salmon
* 1/2 red onion, finely chopped
* 1 bunch of fresh chives, finely chopped
* 2 cloves garlic, peeled and finely chopped
* 1/2-1 tsp Celtic Sea or Himalayan Pink salt and freshly ground black pepper
* 3-4 tbsp rice flour
* 2 tbsp coconut oil

1 Place the salmon fillets in a blender and pulse into chunks, but don't allow it to form a paste.

2 Add the salmon to a large bowl with the rest of the ingredients. Add the rice flour one tablespoon at a time and combine thoroughly. Check the consistency and add a little more to bind the burgers if required. This helps keep them intact while cooking.

3 Heat the coconut oil in a pan over a medium heat. Once the oil has melted, place the burgers in the pan and cook for 4 minutes on each side or until cooked to your liking.

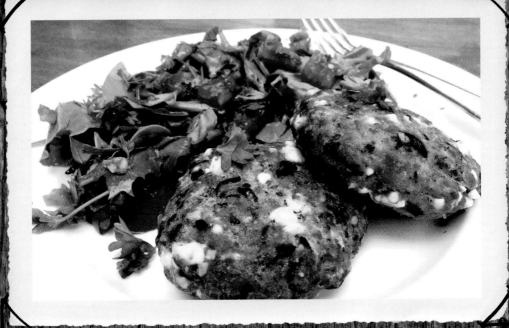

Greek Style Lamb Burgers

Ingredients

* 1 tsp coconut oil
* 1 large handful spinach
* 1 pound (500g) ground lamb
* 2 cloves garlic, peeled and finely chopped
* 5 ounces (150g) feta cheese, crumbled
* 1 handful fresh parsley, chopped
* 2 heaping tsps dried oregano
* 1 handful black olives, chopped
* 1 tbsp olive oil
* Celtic Sea or Himalayan Pink salt and freshly ground black pepper

1 Preheat the oven to 350°F.

2 Heat the coconut oil in a pan and sauté the spinach.

3 Place all the ingredients together in a large bowl and combine thoroughly with your hands.

4 Shape into 4 patties and place on a baking dish or baking tray in the oven to cook for 20-25 minutes.

MAKES:
4 Burgers

PREP TIME
10 Minutes

COOKING TIME
20-25 Minutes

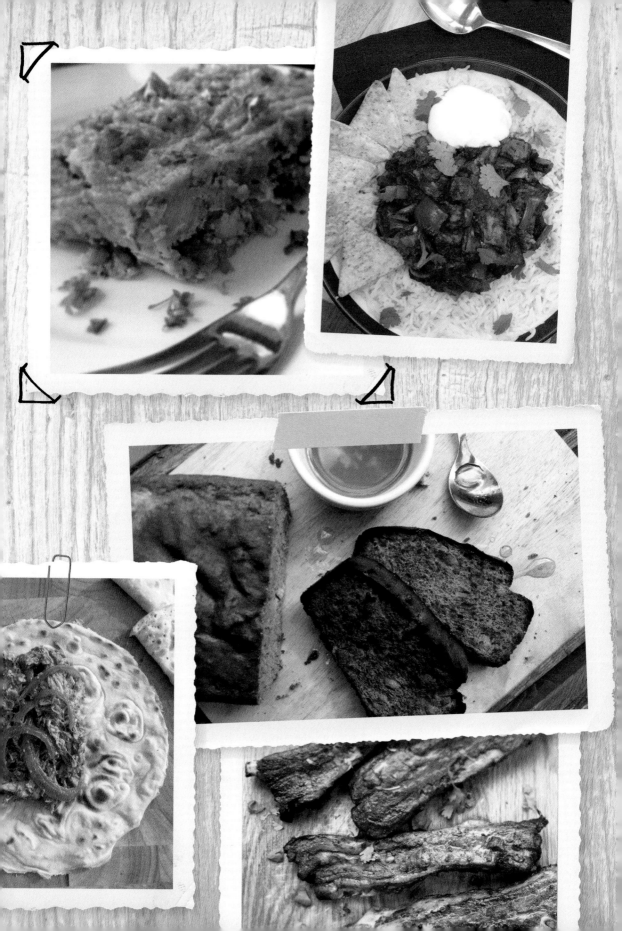

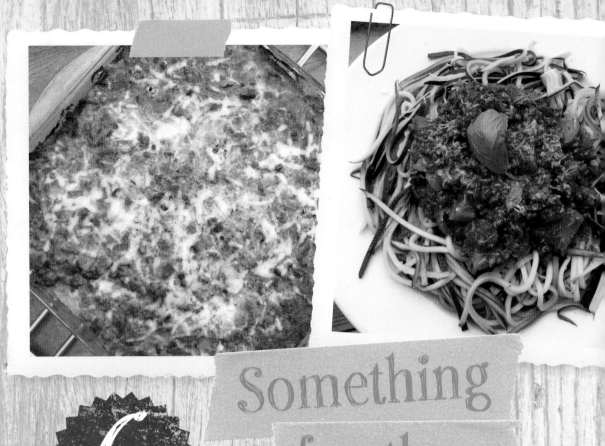

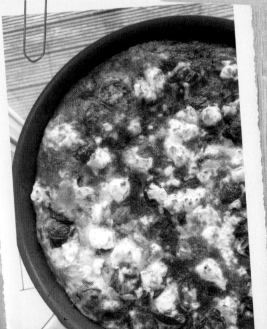

6

Something for the Weekend

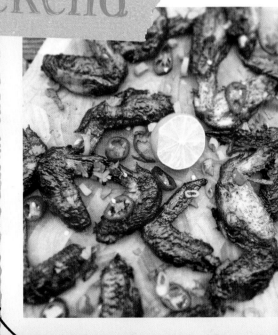

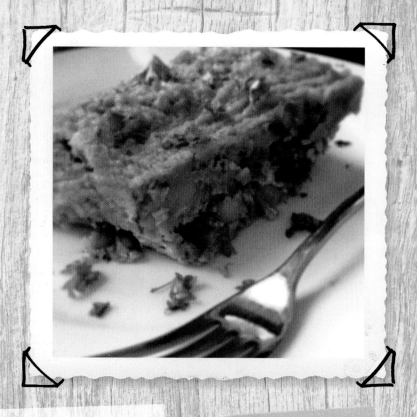

Ingredients

TOPPING

★ 3-4 medium-sized sweet potatoes
   (or white potatoes)
★ 1 tbsp butter (optional)

FISH MIXTURE

★ 1-⅓ pound (600g) fish/seafood
   (white fish, wild salmon, wild shrimp
   or scallops), cut into small 1-inch chunks
★ 1-¾ cups (400ml) coconut milk
★ ¾ pound (350g) carrots, chopped
★ 1 head of broccoli, chopped into
   small florets
★ 2 tsp fresh ginger, grated
★ ½ pound (200g) frozen peas
★ Himalayan Pink or Celtic Sea salt
   and freshly ground black pepper
   to taste

SERVES: 6

**PREP TIME
40 Minutes**

**COOKING TIME
25 Minutes**

Fitter
Fish Pie

1 Preheat the oven to 350°F.

2 Boil or steam the sweet potatoes until they are soft.
Mash for topping the fish pie; add a little butter
if desired.

3 Heat the coconut milk in a saucepan over a
medium heat. When it starts to boil, add the
chopped carrots.

4 Add the fish, peas, ginger and broccoli to the
saucepan and season with salt and pepper.

5 Spoon the fish mixture into an 8-inch Pyrex
oven dish.

6 Spread the mash over the top of the fish mixture
and bake in the oven for 25 minutes.

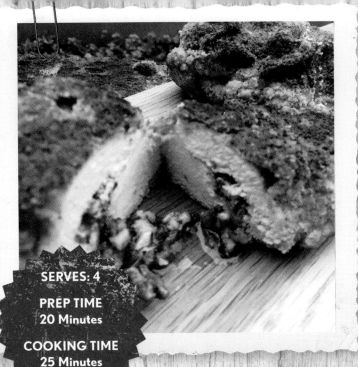
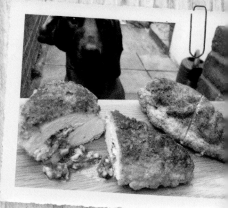

SERVES: 4

PREP TIME
20 Minutes

COOKING TIME
25 Minutes

Chicken Kiev

Ingredients

★ 4 slices smoked bacon
★ Coconut oil or butter for cooking
★ 4 large skinless chicken breasts
★ 3 tbsp rice flour
★ 2 large free-range eggs
★ ¾ cup (150g) ground almonds
★ 1 tsp paprika
★ Himalayan Pink salt and black pepper

FOR THE GARLIC BUTTER

★ 4 cloves garlic, peeled and finely chopped
★ 1 large handful fresh parsley, finely chopped
★ 4 tbsp unsalted butter (at room temperature)
★ ½ tsp cayenne pepper powder

TIP

You can skip the pan frying step if easier. The bacon might not be as crispy and you will need to bake it in the oven for a little longer.

1 Fry the bacon until golden in a pan over a medium heat and set aside.

2 To make the garlic butter, mix the parsley, garlic and cayenne into softened butter and place in the fridge to set. Once set, slice into 4 servings.

3 Cut a little pocket in each chicken breast and stuff with the garlic butter. Crumble one slice of the crispy bacon for each breast and stuff into the breast. Once stuffed, fold and seal the chicken breast, completely covering the butter.

4 Preheat the oven to 350°F.

5 Place the rice flour in a shallow bowl, whisk the eggs in another and place the ground almonds, paprika and a pinch of seasoning into a third.

6 Evenly coat each chicken breast in the rice flour, then roll in the beaten egg, allowing any excess to drip off. Finally coat each piece of chicken in the ground almond mixture.

7 Shallow-fry in ¾-inch of coconut oil or butter over a medium-high heat for 2-3 minutes each side, or until lightly golden. Transfer to a tray and bake in the oven for 15 minutes or until fully cooked.

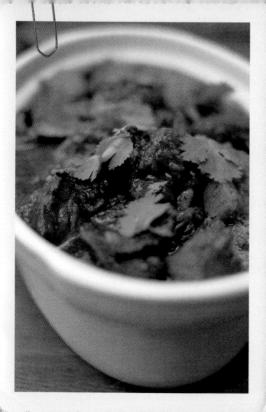

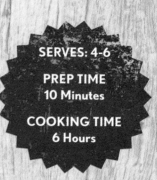

Sweet Potato and Lamb Tagine

Ingredients

★ 2 pounds (1 kg) lamb shoulder, cubed
★ 2 pounds (1 kg) sweet potatoes, peeled and quartered
★ 2-4 tsp Ras el Hanout
★ 1 tsp Celtic Sea or Himalayan Pink salt
★ 2 cloves garlic, peeled and finely chopped
★ 7 ounces (200g) unsulphured apricots
★ 1-½ quarts (1.5 liters) water to cover ingredients

OPTIONAL INGREDIENTS FOR EXTRA SPICE AND FLAVOR

★ 1 tsp ground ginger
★ 1 tsp turmeric
★ 1 tsp black pepper

1 Place the lamb in a large saucepan or slow cooker.

2 Add the sweet potatoes, spices, salt, garlic and apricots.

3 Cover the ingredients with water and simmer over a low heat for 6 hours (or you can bring to a boil and turn down to a medium heat for 2-3 hours).

4 Check the seasoning. If required, add more Ras el Hanout and salt.

5 There is no need to thicken this tagine as the sweet potatoes will disintegrate and thicken the sauce. (If they haven't, mash them a little in the pan before serving.)

TIP

We've also made this recipe with lamb's heart. It's a tasty way of eating organ meats.

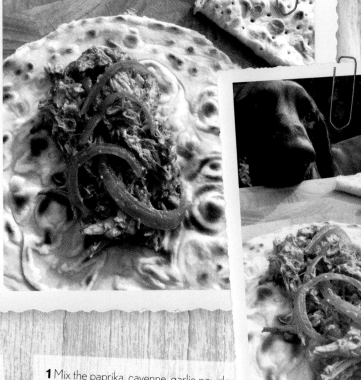

TIP

These are great served in a Breakfast Wrap (see page 93) with crunchy lettuce.

Pulled Pork

Ingredients

★ 4 tbsp paprika or smoked paprika
★ 1-2 tsp cayenne powder (depending on how much kick you like)
★ 2 tsp garlic powder
★ 1 tsp dried thyme
★ 4 tsp Celtic Sea or Himalayan Pink salt
★ 3 tsp freshly ground black pepper
★ 4 tbsp olive oil
★ 4 tbsp apple cider vinegar
★ 4 heaping tbsp honey
★ 2 large onions, peeled and chopped
★ 4 pounds (2 kg) boneless pork shoulder, cut in half and with fat removed (you can use this to make crackling if you wish)

SERVES: 4-6

**PREP TIME
10 Minutes**

**COOKING TIME
8 Hours (check
at 7 Hours)**

1 Mix the paprika, cayenne, garlic powder, thyme, salt and pepper in a bowl with a fork before adding the olive oil, apple cider vinegar and honey and mixing again to form a paste.

2 Place the chopped onion in the bottom of the slow cooker and spread it out before laying the two pieces of pork on top.

3 Pour the paste mixture over the top of the pork, ensuring you use a spoon to get every bit out of the bowl. Then cover as much of the pork as possible with the paste.

4 Turn the slow cooker on to a low setting and cook for 8 hours or until the pork is tender enough to pull apart with a fork.

5 You can either use a fork to shred the pork while it's in the slow cooker and then mix it with the onions and juices, or you can remove the pork from the slow cooker, shred it and then use the onions as a topping.

6 Serve with rice, potatoes or iceberg lettuce wraps.

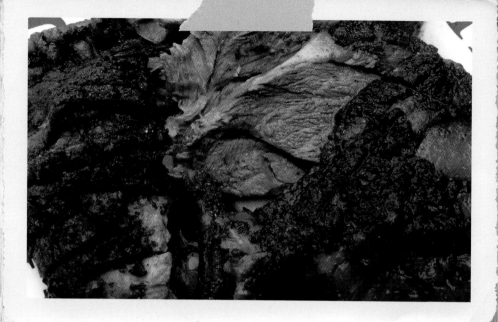

Spicy Roast Shoulder of Lamb

Ingredients

★ 1 whole lamb shoulder
★ 6-7 tbsp olive oil or melted ghee
★ 2 tbsp cumin
★ 2 tbsp cilantro
★ ¾ tsp cinnamon
★ ¼ tsp ground nutmeg
★ Generous pinch of Celtic Sea or Himalayan Pink salt

NOTE

Cooking times for lamb vary depending on both your oven and of course your preference for how you like it cooked. So feel free to modify accordingly.

1 Preheat the oven to 400°F.

2 Mix all the spices and olive oil together in a bowl until it forms a paste. You can add more oil or spices here if you feel you need to.

3 Place the lamb in a baking dish and slash the top with a sharp knife. Cover the top of the lamb with the paste.

4 Place in the oven to cook for 30 minutes until the fat starts to go a little crispy. Then turn the oven down to 350 degrees and cook for another 90 minutes.

5 Remove from the oven and let stand a little before slicing.

6 Pour over the juices from the bottom of the baking tray, and let people help themselves.

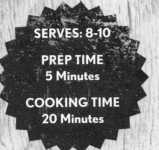

SERVES: 8-10

PREP TIME
5 Minutes

COOKING TIME
20 Minutes

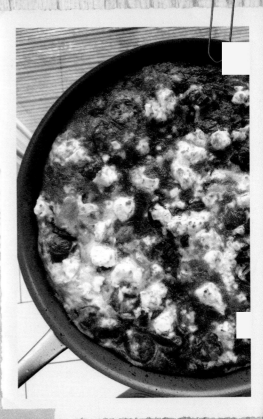

Goat's Cheese, Smoked Salmon and Spinach Frittata

Ingredients

★ 2 tbsp coconut oil, olive oil or butter for cooking
★ 2 cloves garlic, peeled and finely chopped
★ 1 red pepper, deseeded and chopped
★ 4 scallions, chopped
★ 1 large handful cherry tomatoes, halved
★ 2 tsp smoked paprika
★ ½-1tsp cayenne pepper powder
★ Celtic Sea or Himalayan Pink salt and freshly ground black pepper
★ 1 handful broccoli florets, cooked
★ 1 large handful spinach
★ 3-½ ounces (100g) smoked salmon
★ 10-12 eggs, beaten
★ 5 ounces (150g) goat cheese or feta

1 Preheat the broiler.

2 Heat the oil in a pan over medium heat. Add the garlic, peppers, onions and tomatoes and stir fry. Cook for around 4 minutes until the onions and tomatoes begin to soften.

3 Add the paprika, cayenne, salt and pepper, and stir before adding the cooked broccoli and spinach and tossing everything together. Cook until the spinach has wilted down.

4 Stir in the smoked salmon, pour the beaten eggs and crumble the feta over the top.

5 Use a spoon to create little gaps at the bottom of the mixture so the eggs spread as evenly as possible. Allow to cook for a few minutes until the eggs are starting to cook through.

6 Once you can see the base has cooked, remove the pan from the heat and place under the broiler to allow the frittata to fully cook. When the top has turned golden, remove from the broiler and serve.

173

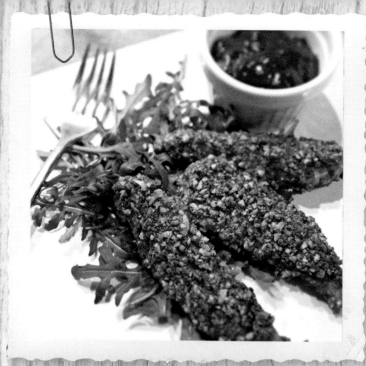

TIP
You can also use a mixture of almonds with gluten-free flour as a coating.

Paprika and Almond Crusted Chicken with Ketchup

Ingredients

★ ¾ pound (350g) chicken breasts
★ 5 ounces (150g) whole blanched almonds
★ 2 tsp paprika or smoked paprika
★ 1 tsp garlic powder
★ ½ tsp Himalayan Pink or Celtic Sea salt
★ 2 egg whites, beaten

SUPER SIMPLE KETCHUP
★ see page 227

1 Preheat the oven to 350°F. Lightly grease a baking tray.

2 Cut the chicken breast in long strips.

3 Place the almonds into a food processor or blender and pulse until they form a breadcrumb-like texture. (Don't blend for too long as you want them to be chunkier than ground almonds.) Sprinkle the almonds onto a plate before adding the paprika, garlic and salt and mixing together well with a fork.

4 Separate the eggs; place the whites into a bowl and whisk.

5 Dip each piece of chicken in the beaten egg white and the roll in the almonds to coat thoroughly. Do this for each piece and place in the prepared baking tray.

6 Bake in the oven for 20-25 minutes. Be careful not to over cook as they will easily burn. Serve with homemade ketchup.

BOSH Bolognese with Zucchini

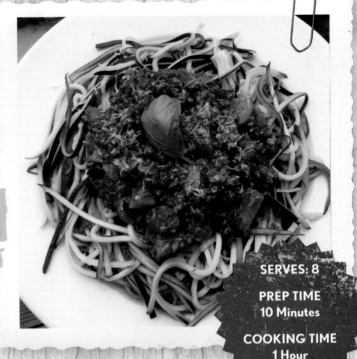

SERVES: 8

PREP TIME
10 Minutes

COOKING TIME
1 Hour

Ingredients

★ 3-½ pounds (1.5 kg) ground lamb
★ 2 tbsp olive oil
★ 6 slices of unsmoked bacon, chopped
★ 4 celery sticks, finely chopped
★ 4 carrots, finely chopped
★ 3 large red onions, peeled
    and finely chopped
★ 6 cloves garlic, peeled
    and finely chopped
★ 3 tbsp mixed herbs
★ 2 tsp paprika
★ 2 sprigs fresh rosemary,
    finely chopped
★ 1 pound (500g) mushrooms,
    finely chopped
★ 4 14-ounce (400g) cans
    chopped tomatoes
★ 6 tbsp tomato purée
★ Celtic Sea or Himalayan Pink salt
    and freshly ground black pepper

TO SERVE
★ Parmigiano cheese
★ Fresh basil leaves

ZUCCHINI
★ 1 zucchini per person for the zucchini
★ Olive oil for cooking

1 Prepare the bolognese sauce by heating the olive oil in a large saucepan over a medium heat, then adding the onions, celery, carrots, bacon and garlic. Stir and cook for around 10 minutes, stirring occasionally until the vegetables start to soften and the bacon has browned a little.

2 Add the ground lamb and stir fry until it begins to brown. Add the mixed herbs, rosemary, paprika, a pinch of salt and some freshly ground pepper. Stir again. Add the tomatoes and purée and combine the ingredients thoroughly. Bring it to a simmer and allow to cook for 45-50 minutes, stirring occasionally. You may wish to add a little water if needed.

3 Around 10 minutes before the bolognese is ready, begin to prepare your zucchini. Heat a little olive oil in a frying pan over a medium heat and use a julienne peeler to slice the zucchini into spaghetti-like strips directly into the pan. One large zucchini is usually enough for one person.

4 Stir fry the zucchini until cooked to your liking. Around 5 minutes is usually enough. Be careful not to overcook as they will turn soggy. Serve the zucchini with the bolognese sauce and top with grated Parmigiano and fresh basil.

NOTE
You will need a nice large saucepan and a julienne peeler for this recipe.

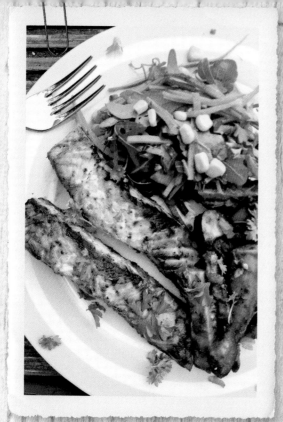

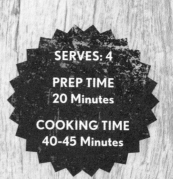

Mediterranean Fish and Chips

Ingredients

- ★ 1 zucchini, chopped
- ★ 1 yellow pepper, chopped
- ★ 1 eggplant, chopped
- ★ 1 tbsp mixed herbs
- ★ 2 cloves garlic, peeled and finely chopped
- ★ 2 sweet potatoes, peeled and chopped into skinny chips/fries
- ★ 4 salmon fillets
- ★ 3 cups (700ml) tomato sauce
- ★ Celtic Sea or Himalayan Pink salt and freshly ground black pepper
- ★ Water

1 Preheat the oven to 350°F.

2 Place the sweet potato chips on a baking tray and set aside.

3 Pour the tomato sauce into a large ovenproof dish. Stir in the herbs salt, pepper, garlic and mix well.

4 Add the chopped zucchini, peppers and eggplant.

5 Combine the ingredients thoroughly in the sauce and place in the oven to bake for 45 minutes.

6 After 20 minutes, place the chips in the oven and lay the salmon fillets on top of the vegetables. Use a spoon to cover the fillets with a little of the sauce. If the sauce is drying, add a little warm water or stock.

7 After 40-45 minutes or until the sweet potatoes and fish are fully cooked, remove from the oven. Place the chips on a plate and top with the salmon and vegetables.

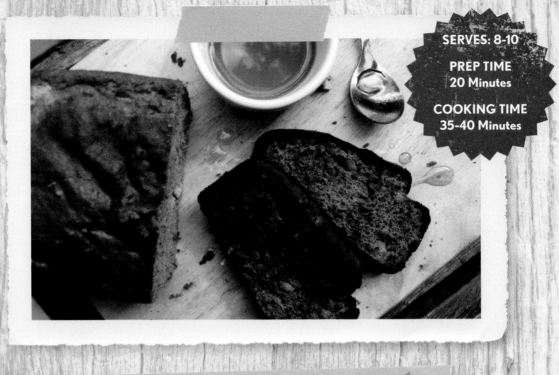

Bacon and Banana Bread with Maple Drizzle

Ingredients

★ 4 bananas
★ 4 eggs
★ 2-3 slices of bacon, chopped
★ 1 tbsp cinnamon
★ ¾ cup (170g) cashew or almond nut butter
★ 2 tbsp unsalted butter or coconut oil
★ 3 Tbsp (50g) coconut flour
★ 1 tsp baking soda
★ 1 tsp gluten-free baking powder
★ 1 tsp vanilla extract

TO SERVE
★ Maple syrup

1 Preheat the oven to 350°F.

2 Line a loaf pan with parchment paper.

3 Chop the banana and add to a food processor with the eggs, nut butter and melted butter (or coconut oil).

4 Sift in the flour, baking powder, cinnamon, baking soda and vanilla extract. Mix until it forms a cake batter. Stir in the chopped bacon. Pour the batter into the lined pan.

5 Bake for 35-40 minutes. Before removing from the oven, insert a knife into the middle and check it comes out clean so you know the loaf is baked all the way through.

6 Once baked, remove from the tin.

7 Serve straight from the oven or toasted with a drizzle of maple syrup.

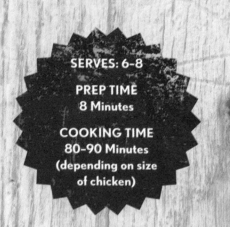

SERVES: 6–8

PREP TIME
8 Minutes

COOKING TIME
80–90 Minutes
(depending on size
of chicken)

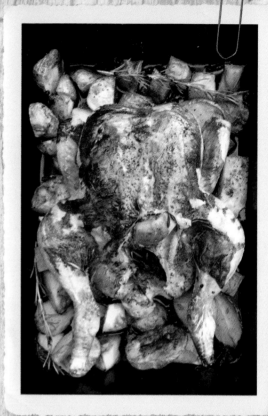

Balsamic
Roast Chicken

Ingredients

★ 1 whole chicken
★ 4 sprigs fresh rosemary
★ 1-¾ pounds (800g) white potatoes
★ 3 tbsp olive oil
★ 8 tbsp balsamic vinegar
★ 3 tbsp honey
★ 1 pack cherry vine tomatoes
   (optional)
★ Celtic Sea or Himalayan Pink salt
   and freshly ground black pepper

1 Preheat the oven to 354°F.

2 Peel the skin away from the chicken breast so you can place sprigs of rosemary underneath.

3 Chop the potatoes and place in a roasting pan with the olive oil and seasoning. Toss together before pushing them to the edges of the pan and placing the chicken in the middle of the pan.

4 Place two more rosemary sprigs inside the chicken and season the skin. Place in the oven to cook for around 1 hour 20 minutes. (Check cooking guidelines per weight of chicken.)

5 Mix the balsamic vinegar and honey together until the honey has dissolved. Once the chicken has been cooking for around 40 minutes, remove it from the oven and pour over the vinegar mix. Place the vine tomatoes around the chicken and put back in the oven to cook for the remaining time.

6 Be sure the chicken is fully cooked, and serve.

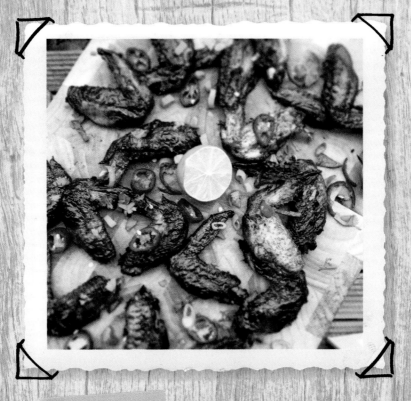

Spicy Ginger Wings

Ingredients

★ 20 chicken wings
★ 4 scallions, finely sliced
★ 1-inch cube fresh ginger, peeled and grated
★ 1 red chili, seeded and finely chopped
★ 1-2 cloves garlic, peeled and finely chopped
★ 4 tbsp honey
★ 2 tbsp tamari
★ Cilantro to garnish

MAKES:
20 wings

PREP TIME
8 Minutes

COOKING TIME
30-35 Minutes

1 Mix all the ingredients except the chicken wings in a large baking dish. Add the wings to the marinade and coat completely.

2 Cover the wings with plastic wrap and leave to marinate for 12-24 hours.

3 Preheat the oven to 480°F.

4 Place the wings in a single llayer on a baking sheet, ensuring all the wings are coated with the marinade. Then place them in the oven and cook for 15 minutes or until they are nice and golden and the skin a little bit crispy. Then turn the oven down to 350°F for 15 more minutes or until fully cooked. Stir occasionally.

5 Remember that cooking times will vary depending on your oven.

6 Top with some chopped scallions, chopped fresh chilies and fresh cilantro, and serve.

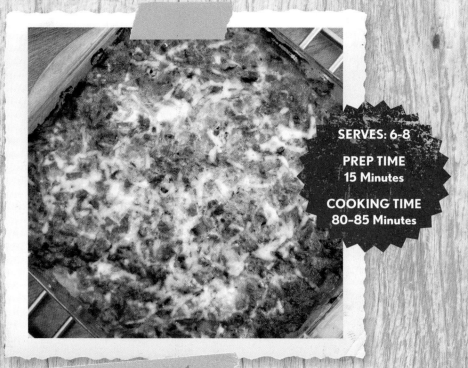

SERVES: 6-8

PREP TIME
15 Minutes

COOKING TIME
80–85 Minutes

Butternut Squash Lasagna

Ingredients

- ★ 2 tbsp olive oil
- ★ 3 cloves of garlic, peeled and finely chopped
- ★ 2 onions, finely chopped
- ★ 2 carrots, sliced then quartered
- ★ ½ pound (250g) mushrooms, sliced
- ★ 1-⅓ pound (600g) ground beef
- ★ 2 tsp oregano
- ★ 2 tsp thyme
- ★ 2 tsp smoked paprika
- ★ Celtic Sea or Himalayan Pink salt and freshly ground black pepper
- ★ 2 14-ounce cans (400g) diced or chopped tomatoes
- ★ 1 medium butternut squash, peeled and sliced around ½ cm thick
- ★ 6 eggs
- ★ ½ cup (100g) cheddar cheese, grated

1 Preheat the oven to 350°F.

2 Heat the olive oil in a large saucepan over medium heat. Add the garlic, onions, carrots, and stir. Cook for 5 minutes or until the onion starts to soften.

3 Add the mushrooms and ground beef and break up the beef as it cooks. Once browned, add the oregano, thyme, smoked paprika, salt and pepper. Stir well and cook for a few minutes. Add the tomatoes and bring to a simmer. Cook for about 30 minutes.

4 Beat the eggs in a bowl and mix with the cheddar cheese.

5 Layer the sliced squash in the base of a baking dish, overlapping the slices a little. Top with a layer of the meat mixture, then cover with half of the egg mix. Top with another layer of squash slices then the rest of the meat, followed by the remaining egg mixture. Give the dish a shake so that the egg runs through all of the gaps.

6 Place in the oven and cook for 50-55 minutes or until the squash is fully cooked.

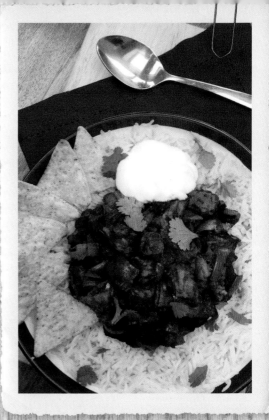

Sweet Potato Chocolate Chili

Ingredients

★ 3-4 medium sweet potatoes, chopped
★ 2 tbsp olive oil for cooking
★ 2-3 tbsp olive oil
★ 1 onion, peeled and chopped
★ 1 green pepper, deseeded and chopped
★ 1 red pepper, deseeded and chopped
★ 1-2 red medium hot chilies, deseeded and finely chopped (depending on how hot you like your chili)
★ 2 cloves of garlic, peeled and finely chopped
★ 1 tsp cayenne pepper powder
★ 1 tsp paprika
★ 1 heaping tsp cumin
★ ½ tsp cinnamon
★ 14-ounce can (400g) cannelli beans or kidney beans (optional, if tolerated)
★ 14-ounce can (400g) chopped tomatoes
★ 1 ounce (30g) dark chocolate (85% cocao)
★ 1 handful fresh cilantro, roughly chopped
★ Celtic Sea or Himalayan Pink salt and freshly ground black pepper

TO SERVE
★ Guacamole, see page 226
★ Plain yogurt or sour cream

1 Preheat the oven to 350°F.

2 Place the potatoes on a baking tray and coat with the olive oil, salt and pepper. Place in the oven for 35-40 minutes or until cooked and slightly crispy around the edges.

3 While the potatoes are cooking, heat some more olive oil in a large pan over a medium heat. Add the onions, peppers, garlic and chilies. Stir and cook for around 5 minutes.

4 Add the cayenne, paprika, cumin and cinnamon. Stir well and cook for a few more minutes before adding the beans and tomatoes.

5 Bring to a boil and then simmer lightly for around 30 minutes, stirring occasionally. If the sauce starts to become too thick, add a little water.

6 Add the chocolate and stir well before adding most of the cilantro (save a little for the topping). Add the sweet potatoes and more seasoning if required, then stir again.

7 Serve topped with the remaining cilantro.

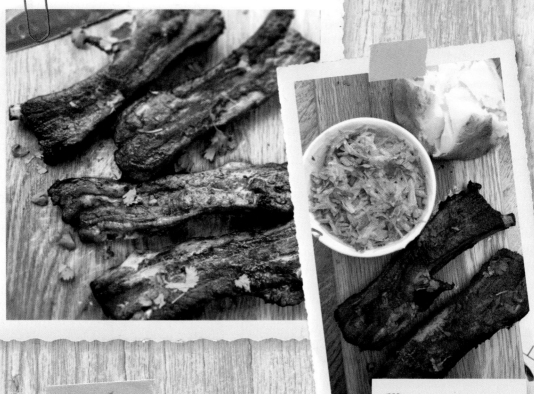

Sticky
Pork Ribs

TIP
These are even tastier if
left to marinate overnight.

Ingredients

★ 6 large pork ribs, scored
★ 1 pound (500g) tomato purée
★ 2 cloves garlic, finely chopped
★ 1-2 tbsp Worcestershire sauce
★ 3 tbsp honey
★ Celtic Sea or Himalayan Pink salt
  and freshly ground black pepper

1 Preheat the oven to 350°F.

2 Place all the ingredients except the ribs in a large bowl
and mix well.

3 Add the ribs and coat thoroughly in the sauce.

4 Place the ribs in a baking tray and pour over the
remaining sauce. Cover with tin foil and place in the
oven to cook for around 30-35 minutes.

5 Remove the foil and cook for another 45-60 minutes.
Turn the ribs over half way through the
cooking time.

MAKES:
6 Ribs

PREP TIME
5 Minutes

COOKING TIME
80-90 Minutes

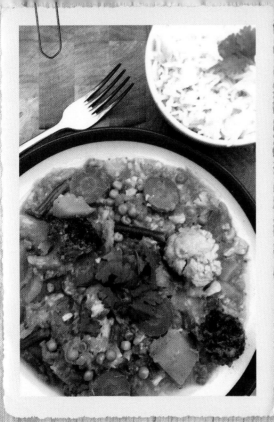

SERVES: 8-10

PREP TIME
20 Minutes

COOKING TIME
55-60 Minutes

Veggie Fest Curry

Ingredients

★ 1 tsp coconut oil
★ 3 cloves garlic
★ 1 white onion, peeled and chopped
★ 1 large chunk of ginger, chopped and peeled
★ 2 tbsp medium curry powder
★ 1 small butternut squash, peeled and cubed
★ 5 carrots, sliced
★ 18-ounce can (500ml) coconut milk
★ ½ cup (100g) creamed coconut bar (optional: makes a richer curry)
★ 1 broccoli floret
★ 1 small cauliflower
★ ½ pound (250g) peas
★ Celtic Sea or Himalayan Pink salt and freshly ground black pepper
★ Water

1 Place the coconut oil in a large casserole dish over a medium heat.

2 Stir fry the onions, garlic, ginger and curry powder for 5 minutes

3 Add the squash, carrots and coconut milk, and bring to a simmer.

4 Add the creamed coconut bar if using.

5 Stir and allow to simmer for 35-40 minutes until the squash is soft.

6 Finally add the broccoli, cauliflower and peas, and cook for another 10 minutes. If the mixture is too thick, add a little boiling water.

7 Season to taste and serve.

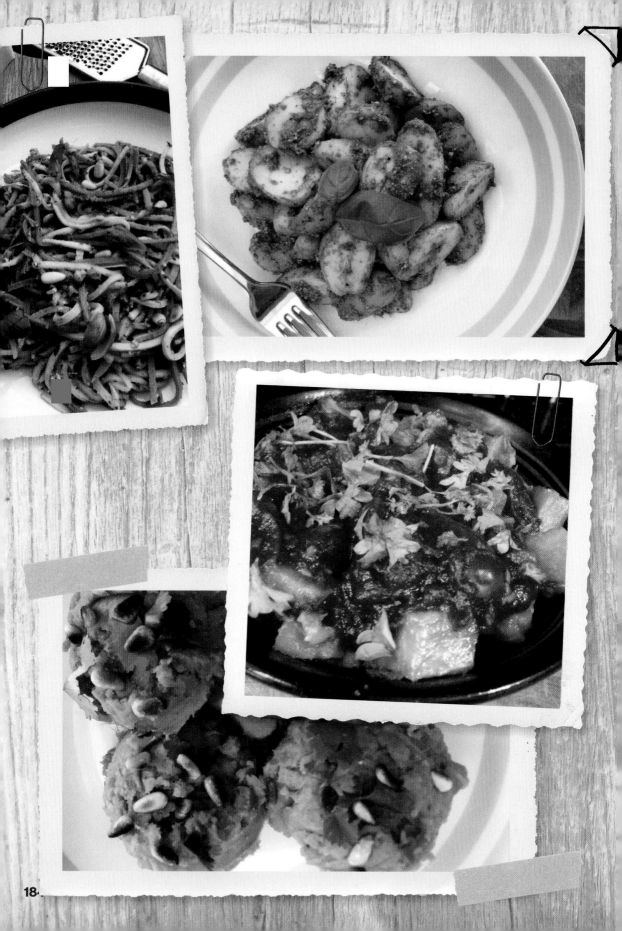

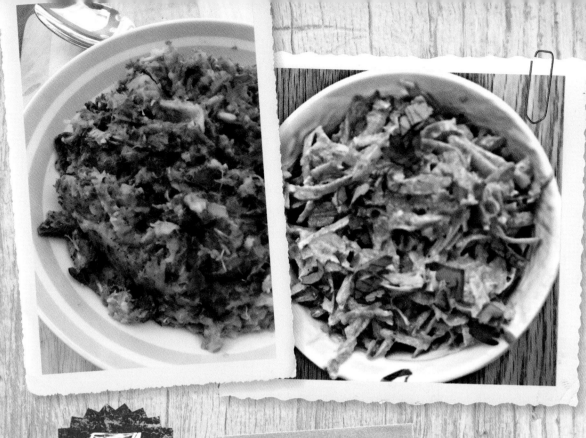

7

Sides

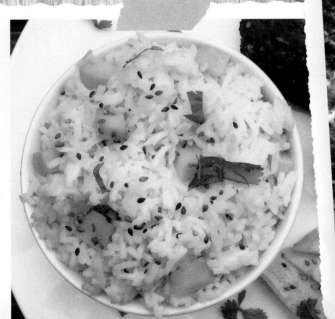

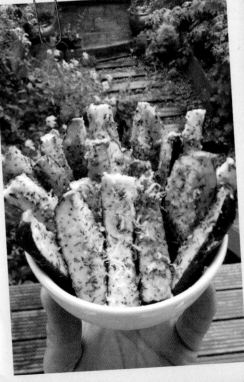

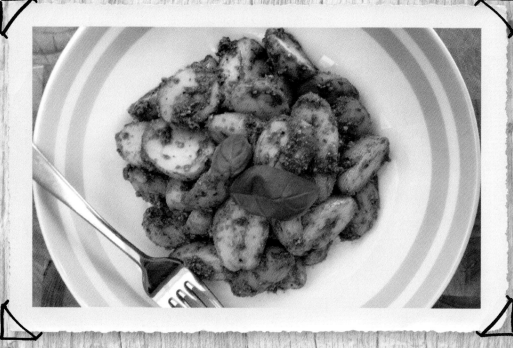

Pimped Up Pesto Potatoes

SERVES: 4

PREP TIME
6 Minutes

COOKING TIME
12 Minutes

Ingredients

★ Large handful fresh basil
★ 1 ripe Hass avocado, peeled, halved and stone removed
★ 1-2 garlic cloves, crushed
★ ¼ cup (50g) walnuts, roasted or lightly toasted (pine nuts, macadamia nuts or cashews work well too)
★ Juice of 1 lemon
★ 1 tbsp olive oil
★ Celtic Sea or Himalayan Pink salt and freshly ground black pepper
★ 1 pound (500g) new potatoes, halved
★ 3-½ ounces (100g) cherry tomatoes, halved
★ Fresh basil to garnish

1 Place the new potatoes in a steamer or in some simmering lightly salted water to cook for about 8-10 minutes or until soft.

2 While they cook, prepare your pesto by placing the basil, garlic, avocado, olive oil, lemon juice, nuts, salt and pepper into a blender and mix for about 20-30 seconds. Feel free to add a little water if you prefer a thinner consistency. Taste and add more basil or seasoning if you wish.

3 When the potatoes are finished cooking, drain them and add them to a heated pan. Then add the pesto and cherry tomatoes and stir well until the potatoes are fully coated and the pesto has heated.

4 Serve topped with fresh basil and you're good to go.

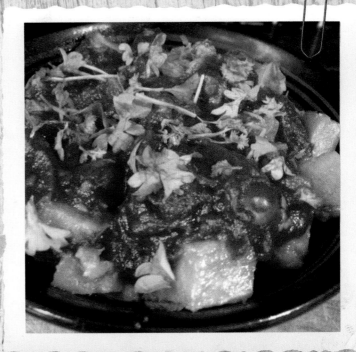

Sweet Patatas Bravas

Ingredients

★ 4 medium sweet potatoes, chopped into cubes (use white potatoes if you prefer)
★ ⅔ pound tomato purée (300g)
★ 1 medium sized onion, peeled and finely chopped
★ 3 tomatoes, finely chopped
★ 2 garlic cloves, crushed or finely chopped
★ 2 tsp smoked paprika (reduce or increase depending on taste)
★ Pinch of cayenne pepper powder (reduce or increase depending on taste)
★ 1 tbsp coconut oil or butter for cooking
★ Himalayan Pink salt or Celtic Sea salt
★ 1 handful fresh parsley

SERVES: 2

PREP TIME
5 Minutes

COOKING TIME
30 Minutes

1 Preheat the oven to 350°F.

2 Melt the coconut oil or butter in a baking dish and add the sweet potato (save a little oil for the sauce). Give it a stir to ensure the potatoes are fully coated in the oil, sprinkle with salt and place in the oven.

3 Leave these to cook for about 25 minutes or until soft. Stir occasionally.

4 When your potatoes are half way through the cooking time, start to prepare the sauce.

5 Add the remaining coconut oil to a saucepan over a medium heat and then add the garlic and onion. Cook until they start to soften, then add the tomato purée, tomatoes, smoked paprika, cayenne powder, a little salt and then stir well. Simmer for about 10 minutes, stirring occasionally.

6 Once the potatoes are fully cooked, remove from the oven, place in a bowl, top with the sauce and sprinkle a generous handful of fresh parsley over the top.

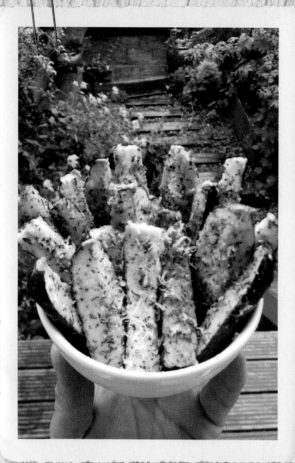

SERVES: 2

PREP TIME
5 Minutes

COOKING TIME
12-15 Minutes

Cheesy Zucchini Chips

Ingredients

★ 2 Tbsp (30-40g) parmesan cheese, grated
★ 1 tsp oregano
★ 1 tsp thyme
★ ½ tsp garlic powder
★ 2 tbsp olive oil
★ Celtic Sea or Himalayan Pink salt and freshly ground black pepper
★ 4 medium zucchini, quartered length ways

1 Preheat the oven to 350°F.

2 Mix the parmesan, oregano, thyme, garlic, salt and pepper together and place on a plate.

3 Pour the olive oil onto a baking tray.

4 Place each zucchini chip in the olive oil to coat a little and then dip in the cheese mixture. Place skin side down on the baking tray. Repeat for each zucchini chip, and then sprinkle the remaining mixture over the top.

5 Place in the oven to cook for 12-15 minutes.

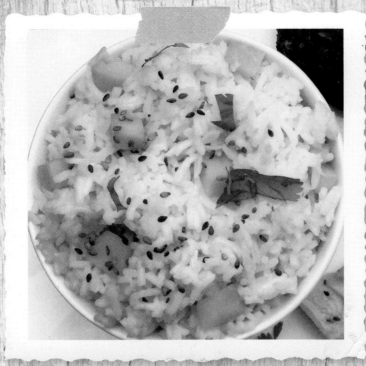

Sticky Coconut Mango Rice

Ingredients
★ 1 pat of butter
★ 1 pack quick cook basmati rice
★ 5-ounce can (150ml) coconut milk
★ 2 tsp desiccated coconut
★ 1 small mango, peeled and chopped
   into small cubes
★ 1 tsp sesame seeds

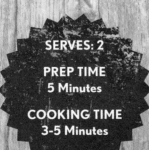

SERVES: 2

PREP TIME
5 Minutes

COOKING TIME
3-5 Minutes

1 Melt the butter in a saucepan on medium heat before adding the rice and stirring well.

2 As the butter is melting, heat a frying pan over a medium heat and add the sesame seeds to the pan without oil to cook for a few minutes until golden.

3 Shake the coconut milk in the can, open and stir. Add to the saucepan and stir again. Cook for 2-3 minutes.

4 Add the desiccated coconut and the mango chunks, and stir well. Cook for another minute or so until it has a nice creamy texture.

5 Top with the sesame seeds and serve.

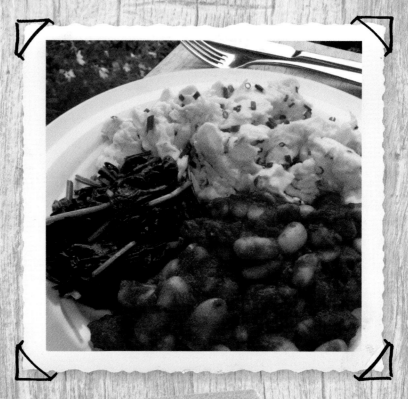

BOSH
Baked Beans

Ingredients

- ★ 1–2 tbsp olive oil
- ★ 3 cloves garlic, peeled and finely chopped
- ★ 2 14-ounce cans (400g) chopped tomatoes
- ★ 4 tbsp Worcestershire sauce
- ★ Celtic Sea or Himalayan Pink salt and freshly ground black pepper
- ★ 14-ounce can (400g) butter beans, drained
- ★ 14-ounce can (400g) cannellini beans, drained

1 Heat the olive oil in a pan over a medium heat. Add the garlic and cook for a couple of minutes. (Do not burn.)

2 Add the tomatoes and Worcestershire sauce, and stir well. Bring to a simmer and cook for 6 minutes.

3 Add the beans, stir well and cook for another 6–8 minutes, stirring occasionally.

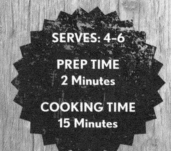

SERVES: 4–6

PREP TIME
2 Minutes

COOKING TIME
15 Minutes

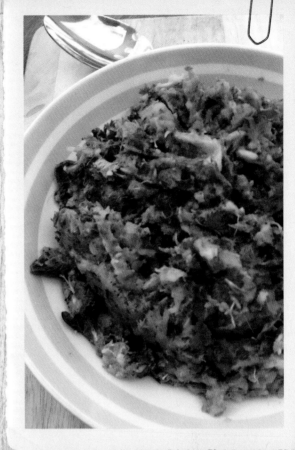

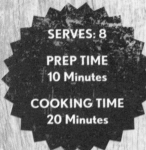

Super Mash

Ingredients

★ 1-⅓ pound (600g) white potatoes, peeled and chopped
★ 1-⅓ pound (600g) sweet potatoes, peeled and chopped
★ 1 large leek, chopped
★ 4 cloves of garlic, peeled and finely chopped
★ 2-inch cube of fresh ginger, peeled and finely chopped
★ ⅔ pound (300g) broccoli florets
★ Large handful kale, chopped
★ Large handful spinach
★ 1/2 pound (290g) sun-dried tomatoes in olive oil
★ Celtic Sea or Himalayan Pink salt and freshly ground black pepper

TO SERVE
★ Fresh parsley

1 Place the potatoes and leeks into a steamer and top with the chopped garlic and ginger before covering. Cook for around 15 minutes or until the potatoes are soft.

2 Just before the potatoes are ready, steam the broccoli, kale and spinach for 5-7 minutes.

3 Drain the cooked potatoes and vegetables, and place in a large bowl. Add the sun-dried tomatoes, including the olive oil as this adds lots of flavor. Add the salt and pepper and mash everything together until it reaches the desired consistency.

4 Serve with fresh parsley.

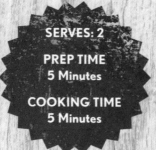

SERVES: 2

PREP TIME
5 Minutes

COOKING TIME
5 Minutes

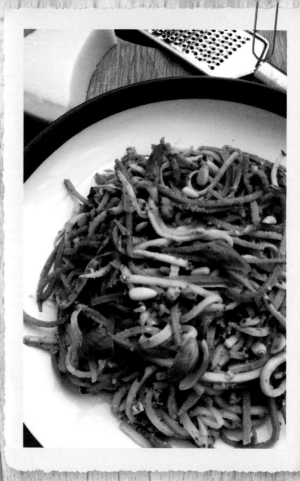

Pesto Veghetti

Ingredients

FOR THE PESTO
★ 2 tbsp olive oil
★ A couple of large handfuls fresh basil
★ 1 clove garlic, peeled
★ 2 tbsp Parmesan, finely grated
★ 1 handful lightly toasted pine nuts
★ Celtic Sea or Himalayan Pink salt
   and freshly ground black pepper
★ 1–2 tsp lemon juice

FOR THE VEGHETTI
★ 1 tbsp olive oil
★ 2 zucchini, julienned
★ 2 carrots, julienned

1 Place all the pesto ingredients in a food processor and blend into a thick, creamy consistency. Add more olive oil if required. Blend just enough so the pine nuts are still a little intact to add crunch to the pesto.

2 Heat the olive oil in a pan over a medium heat. Add the zucchini and carrots and give them a stir, cooking for a couple of minutes.

3 Stir the pesto in with the vegetables and coat fully. Cook for another 2–3 minutes.

4 Top with some more pine nuts, fresh basil and a little Parmesan if desired.

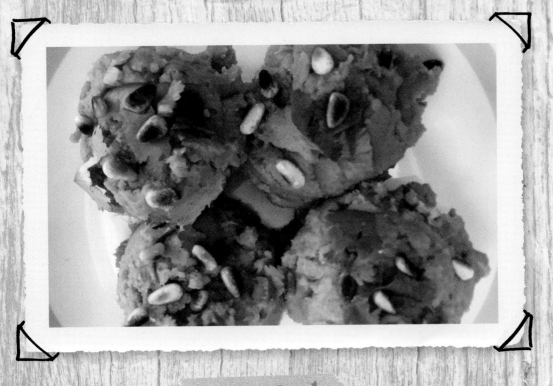

Curried
Sweet Potato Mash

Ingredients

★ 2-3 medium sweet potatoes, peeled and chopped
★ 2-3 tsp medium curry powder
★ 1 tsp garlic powder
★ 1 handful fresh cilantro, roughly chopped
★ Celtic Sea or Himalayan Pink salt and freshly ground black pepper
★ 2-3 tbsp pine nuts (optional)

1 Place the sweet potatoes in a steamer and cook until soft.

2 Place in a large bowl and add the curry powder, garlic, fresh cilantro, salt and pepper.

3 Place the pine nuts in a dry pan over a medium heat to toast lightly while you mash the potatoes.

4 Top the potatoes with the toasted pine nuts and fresh cilantro to serve.

SERVES: 2-4

PREP TIME
5 Minutes

COOKING TIME
15 Minutes

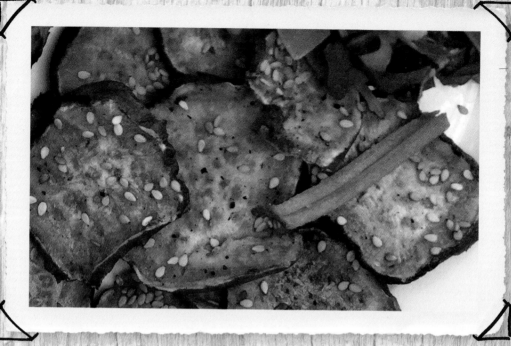

Crinkle Cut Sesame Sweet Pot Chips

Ingredients

★ 2-3 medium sized sweet potatoes
★ 2-3 tbsp olive oil
★ 3 tsp sesame seeds
★ Celtic Sea or Himalayan Pink salt and freshly ground black pepper

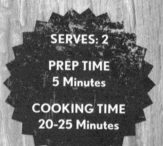

SERVES: 2

PREP TIME
5 Minutes

COOKING TIME
20-25 Minutes

1 Preheat the oven to 350°F.

2 Using a crinkle cutter, cut the sweet potatoes thinly; less than ¼-inch if you can.

3 Spread the olive oil on a baking tray and spread out the sweet potato slices out in a single layer.

4 Coat both sides with a little oil before topping with sesame seeds, salt and pepper.

5 Place in the oven and cook until crispy round the edges.

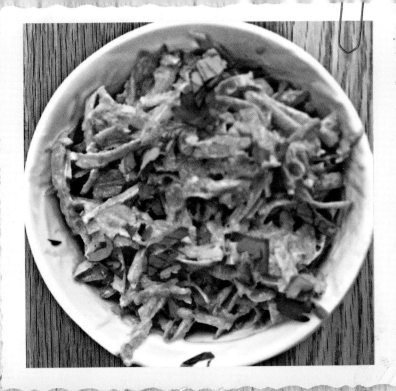

Quick
Carrot and Cilantro
Slaw

Ingredients

★ 1 large or 2 medium carrots, grated
★ 2 heaping tbsp Greek yogurt
★ 1 tsp honey
★ 1 handful fresh cilantro, roughly
    chopped
★ Freshly ground black pepper

1 Mix the yogurt and honey together thoroughly in a bowl.

2 Stir in the grated carrot, fresh cilantro and black pepper, and mix together thoroughly.

3 Top with some fresh cilantro and serve.

SERVES: 2

PREP TIME
3 Minutes

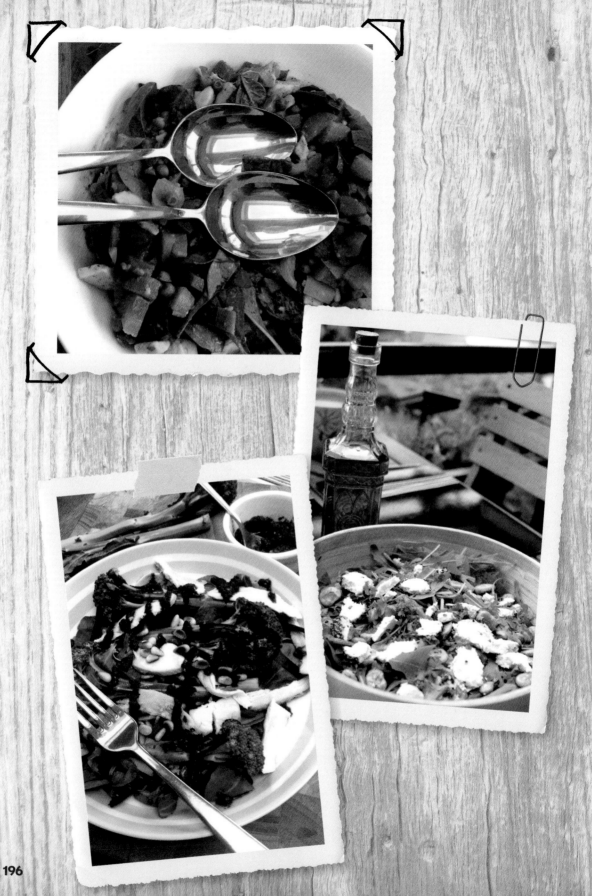

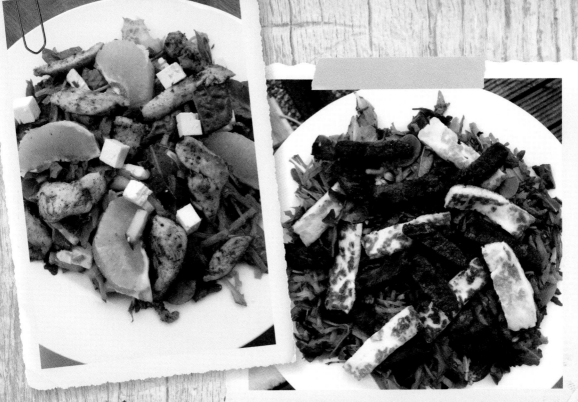

8 Salads

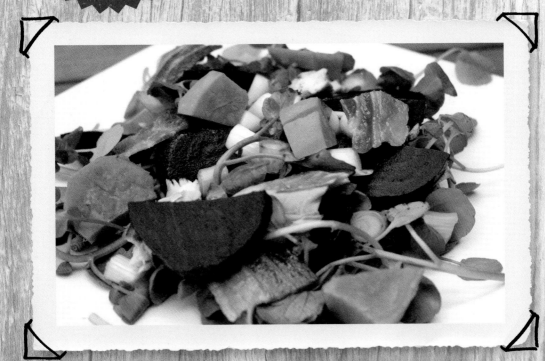

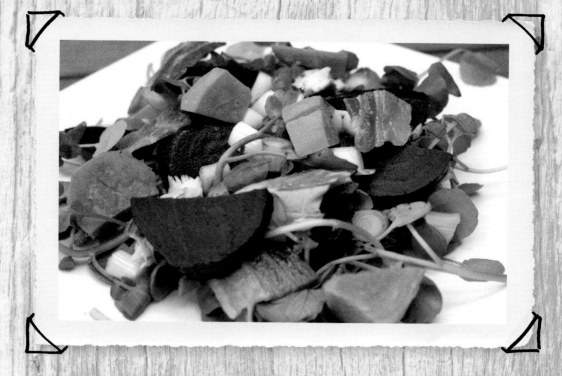

How to
Pimp a Salad

To really '**pimp**' a salad, follow this simple 3-step process:

1 Choose a base.
2 Choose a taste.
3 Stuff it in your face. ☺

Choose a base

Green stuff is highly nutritious—fact! Green leafy vegetables are a rich source of vitamins and antioxidants. Where possible, purchase organic and local. Some of the most nutritious greens include:

★ Kale
★ Spinach
★ Red lettuce
★ Arugula
★ Watercress

★ Mustard greens
★ Chard
★ Purslane
★ Radicchio
★ Romaine

Choose a Taste

The most nutritious salad greens can be a little bitter, so it's essential to add some extra flavors to complement the taste and get you more excited about eating garden! The possibilities are endless...

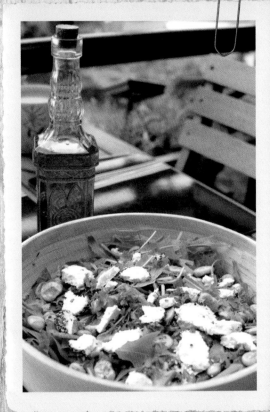

★ Freshly squeezed lemon or lime juice
★ Apple cider vinegar (unpasteurized has the most nutritional benefits)
★ Pumpkin seeds dried in the oven and tossed in chili or cayenne pepper
★ Soaked and baked walnuts, hazelnuts or cashews
★ Seaweed sprinkles or flakes
★ Avocado
★ Sun-dried tomatoes
★ Grated carrot
★ Sliced beets
★ Olives
★ Celtic Sea salt or Himalayan Pink salt
★ Cracked black pepper
★ Jalapenos
★ Fresh mint leaves
★ Fresh cilantro
★ Fresh basil
★ Strawberries (yes, really!)
★ Eggs: boiled, poached, fried
★ Capers
★ Bacon ☺ **Matt's Favorite**
★ Roasted cherry tomatoes
★ Julienned zucchini
★ Fresh peas ☺ **Keris's Favorite**
★ Roasted butternut squash
★ Pancetta
★ Pine nuts
★ Dried mixed herbs
★ Crushed chilies

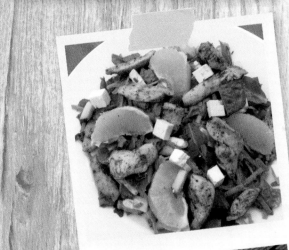

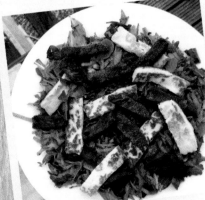

Now... Stuff it in your face. ☺

199

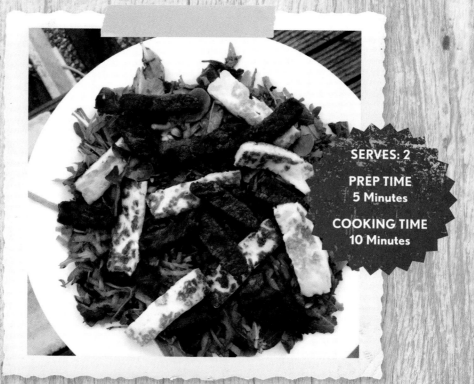

Steak and Halloumi Salad

Ingredients

★ 2 handfuls spinach
★ 2 handfuls arugula
★ 1 handful grated carrot
★ 1 handful cherry tomatoes, quartered
★ 2 tbsp olive oil
★ 2 8-ounce (250g) steaks, cut into strips
★ 2 tsp smoked paprika
★ 1 tsp garlic powder
★ ½-1 tsp cayenne pepper powder
★ Celtic Sea or Himalayan Pink salt and freshly ground black pepper
★ 3 ounce (80g) halloumi cheese, sliced

TO SERVE
★ Drizzle of olive oil

1 Place the spinach, arugula, carrot and tomatoes in a large bowl and toss together.

2 Heat 1 tablespoon of the olive oil in a pan over a medium heat before adding the steak strips and cooking for around a minute or until the steak browns slightly. Add the paprika, garlic powder, cayenne, salt and pepper. Stir and cook for about 6-8 minutes or until the steak is cooked to your liking.

3 When the steak is nearly done, heat the remaining olive oil in another pan and add the halloumi slices. Cook for a couple of minutes on each side or until golden.

4 Divide the salad into two serving bowls and top with the steak strips. Slice the halloumi lengthways and add to the salad.

5 Drizzle with olive oil and serve.

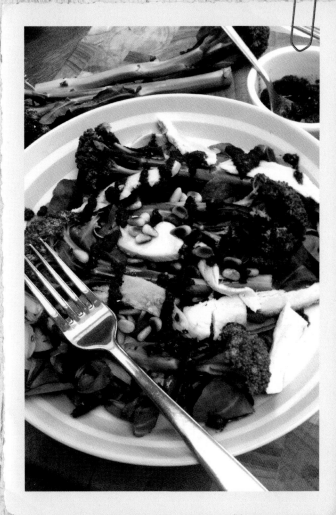

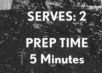

Goji Green Salad

Ingredients
★ 2 large handfuls mixed greens salad
★ 2 tbsp Homemade Pesto*
   (see page 228) *save some
   toasted pine nuts to top the salad
★ 2 tbsp goji berries
★ 6 stalks broccolini,
   lightly steamed
★ 8 ounces (200-300g) cooked
   chicken or turkey, chopped
★ Celtic Sea or Himalayan Pink salt
   and freshly ground black pepper

1 Add the salad leaves, broccolini, goji berries and chicken/turkey to a large salad bowl and toss together.

2 Pour over the homemade pesto, top with pine nuts and serve.

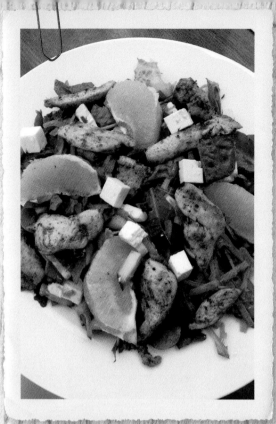

SERVES: 2

PREP TIME
5 Minutes

COOKING TIME
7–10 Minutes

Chicken, Cumin and Orange Salad

Ingredients

★ 2 large handfuls mixed greens salad
★ 2 grated carrots
★ Half a cucumber, chopped
★ Zest of half an orange
★ Juice of an orange
★ 2 tbsp olive oil
★ 1 tsp cumin seeds
★ 4 ounces (100g) feta cheese, chopped
★ 1 tbsp coconut oil
★ 2 chicken breasts, chopped
★ ½-1 tsp garlic powder
★ 1 tsp cumin powder
★ Celtic Sea or Himalayan Pink salt
   and freshly ground black pepper
★ 1 orange, sliced then skin removed
   (much neater than peeling first!)

1 Add the salad leaves, carrots, cucumber, orange zest and juice, olive oil, cumin seeds and feta to a large salad bowl and toss together.

2 Heat the coconut oil in a pan on a medium heat and then add the chicken.

3 Cook the chicken for about a minute, and add the garlic, cumin, salt and pepper, and stir together. Continue to cook the chicken for another 6–8 minutes or until cooked.

4 Serve the salad topped with the chicken and orange slices. Add a little more feta if you fancy—and enjoy.

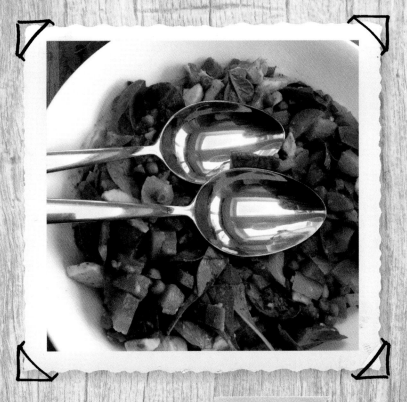

Ingredients

★ 3 large carrots, chopped into small
  chunks
★ 7 ounces (200g) peas
★ 1 yellow pepper, deseeded and
  chopped into chunks
★ 1 avocado, skin removed and
  chopped into small chunks
★ 2-3 handfuls baby spinach
  or arugula leaves
★ Handful fresh mint
★ Handful fresh parsley
★ 1 handful fresh cilantro
★ 2 tbsp olive oil
★ 2 tbsp apple cider vinegar
★ Celtic Sea or Himalayan Pink salt
  and freshly ground black pepper
★ 1 clove garlic, peeled
★ Juice of 1 lemon

TO SERVE
★ Crumbled feta or pan-fried fish
  or chicken (optional)

Epic Herby Salad

1 Steam or boil the carrots, peas and pepper until soft.

2 Place the cooked vegetables in a bowl and stir in the avocado and salad leaves.

3 Place the herbs, garlic, oil, lemon juice and vinegar in a blender and combine into a creamy dressing. Pour over the salad and toss the ingredients to coat the vegetables in the dressing.

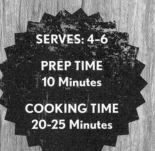

SERVES: 4–6

**PREP TIME
10 Minutes**

**COOKING TIME
20-25 Minutes**

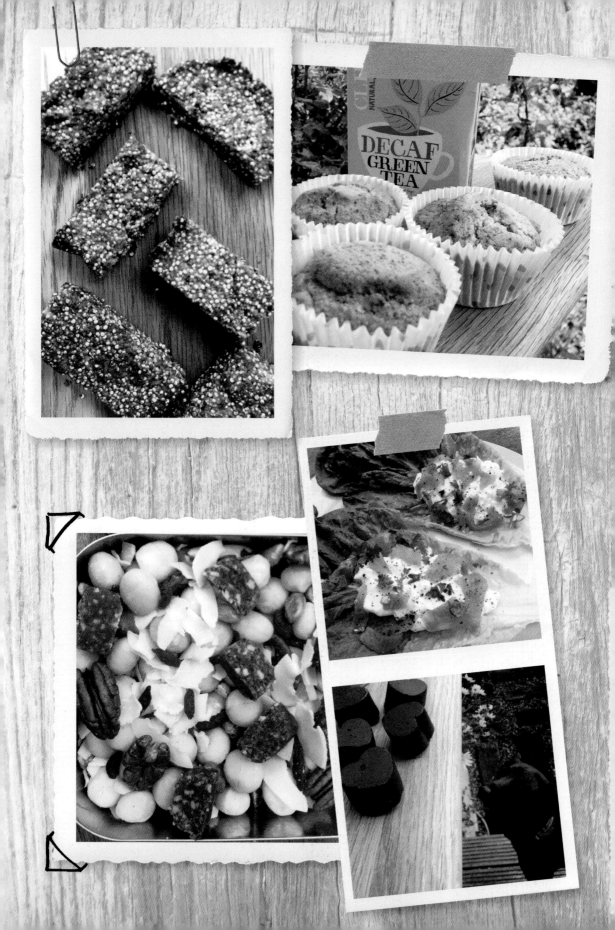

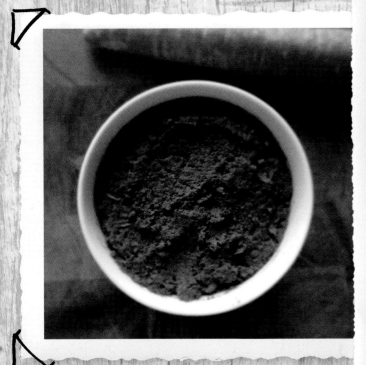

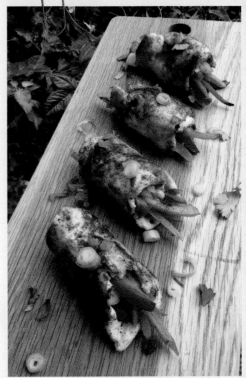

9

Snacks & Superfoods

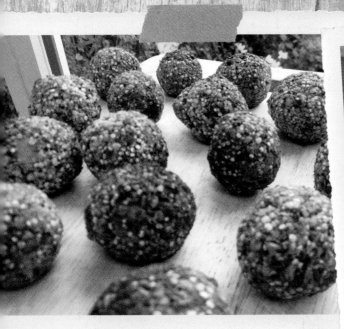

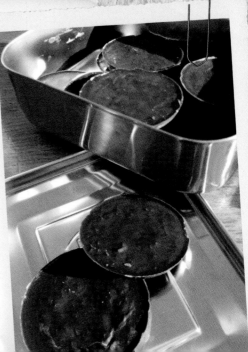

Snack Inspiration

The following don't really qualify as recipes; they're just designed to inspire you to pimp your snacks:

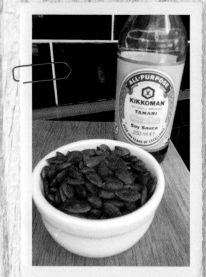

Tamari Nuts and Pumpkin Seeds

Sprinkle nuts with tamari sauce and bake in the oven for 10-15 minutes on 350°F.

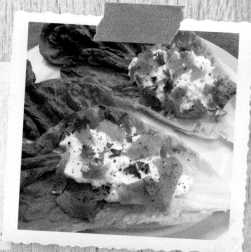

Lettuce Wraps

Get some large romaine lettuce leaves and serve with your favorite sandwich fillers. Try the following:
★ Salmon and cottage cheese
★ Bacon and avocado
★ Tuna and eggs
★ Parma ham and sundried tomatoes

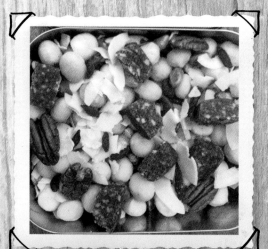

Fitter Trail Mix

Mixed nuts, seeds, coconut chips and goji berries with some chopped fruit bars or your favorite protein bars.

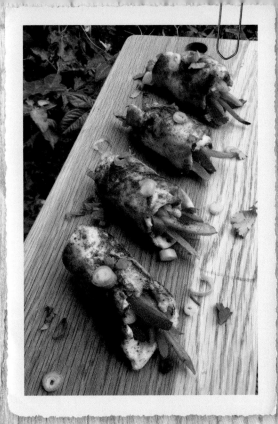

Chicken Squids

Ingredients

★ 2 chicken breasts
★ ½ tsp garlic powder
★ ½ tsp smoked paprika
★ ¼ tsp cayenne pepper powder (optional)
★ Himalayan Pink or Celtic Sea salt and freshly ground black pepper
★ ½ red pepper, thinly sliced lengthways
★ ½ green pepper, thinly sliced lengthways
★ 1 carrot, sliced into thin sticks
★ 1 scallions, chopped
★ 1 handful fresh cilantro
★ 2 tbsp coconut oil

1 Place each chicken breast between two sheets of plastic wrap, and using a rolling pin or meat hammer give the chicken a good wallop until both chicken breasts are nice and flat. (Not so much that they split!)

2 Cut the breasts down the middle lengthways so you now have four pieces. Then sprinkle each piece evenly with the paprika, garlic, cayenne, salt and pepper.

3 Divide the peppers and carrots evenly between the four pieces and place them in the chicken, across the middle. Top each with the scallions and cilantro before wrapping the chicken around the veg like a fajita wrap. You will need a toothpick to stick through to keep it together.

4 Heat the oil in a pan on a medium heat before adding each little wrap. Sprinkle them with a little more paprika and garlic before cooking for about 8-10 minutes, turning occasionally so they are golden brown all over.

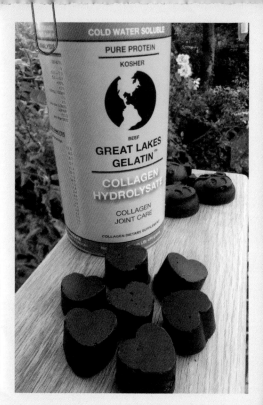

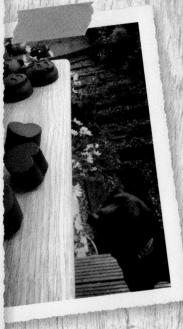

Chocolate
Collagen Bites

SUPERFOOD

Ingredients
★ 7 ounces (200g) 85-90% dark
  chocolate, melted
★ 1 ounce (30g) goji berries
★ ¾ ounce (20g) cacao nibs
★ Pinch of Himalayan Pink
  or Celtic Sea salt
★ 2 ounces (50g) hydrolysed collagen

1 Prepare some chocolate molds by placing on a baking tray (so they are easy to transfer into the fridge).

2 Place the melted chocolate in a mixing bowl and add the goji berries, cacao nibs, salt and collagen, and combine thoroughly.

3 Pour the mixture into the chocolate molds.

4 Place in the fridge to set for one hour.

MAKES:
14-16 Chocolates

PREP TIME
10 Minutes

Bone Broth

A hug in a mug

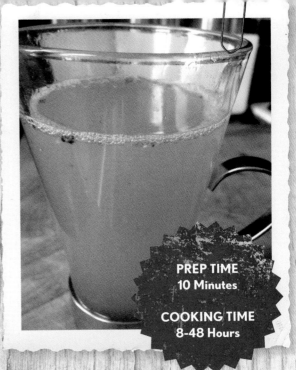

When selecting bones for your broth, always try to source them from grass-fed animals or free-range, pastured poultry. Soaking the bones and cooking them for long periods of time creates a broth rich in proteins and minerals. Places to find good bones include:

★ From a local butcher, especially one who butchers the whole animal

★ From local farmers who raise grass-fed animals (ask at your local farmer's market)

PREP TIME
10 Minutes

COOKING TIME
8-48 Hours

Ingredients
★ 2-½ pounds of bones
★ 1 onion
★ 2 carrots
★ 2 stalks of celery
★ 2 tbsp apple cider vinegar
★ 2 cloves garlic
★ Filtered water

OPTIONAL
★ 1 tbsp Celtic Sea or Himalayan Pink salt
★ 1 tsp peppercorns
★ Additional herbs or spices to taste, e.g. rosemary, thyme or dried mixed herbs

TO SERVE (OPTIONAL)
★ 2-3 organic egg yolks (these gently poach in hot broth or you can stir them in to make a creamy broth).

You will need a large casserole pot or slow cooker to cook the broth in, and a sieve to remove the pieces when it's done.

1 Place the bones in a large stock pot. Pour (filtered) water over the bones and add the vinegar. Allow to sit for 20-30 minutes in the cool water. The acid from the vinegar helps to make the nutrients in the bones more available.

2 Roughly chop and add the vegetables to the pot. Add any salt, pepper, spices or herbs, if using.

3 Bring the broth to a boil and then reduce to a simmer. If using a slow cooker, set to low heat. These are suggested times to cook the bones:
★ Beef broth/stock: 24-48 hours
★ Chicken or poultry broth/stock: 24 hours
★ Fish broth: 8 hours

4 Remove from the heat and allow to cool slightly. Strain using a sieve to remove all the bones, fat and vegetables.

5 Store in a glass jar or bowl in the fridge. The fat will set on top and can be scooped off and kept for cooking vegetables.

6 Broth will keep for up to 5 days, or you can freeze it for later use.

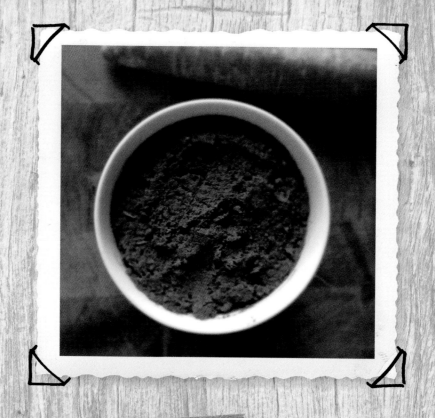

Dairy-free Liver Paté

Ingredients

★ 14 ounces (400g) liver (we used chicken liver for this, but you can try lamb's or calf's liver)
★ 8 slices of unsmoked bacon, cut into small pieces
★ ½ onion, finely chopped
★ 2 egg yolks
★ 1 tsp mixed herbs
★ 1 tbsp fresh rosemary, finely chopped
★ Freshly ground black pepper

SERVES: 3-4

PREP TIME
10 Minutes

COOKING TIME
20 Minutes

1 Pan fry the liver in coconut oil over medium heat for 10 minutes or until cooked to your liking, then set aside to cool.

2 Pan fry the onions and bacon in coconut oil over medium heat for 8–10 minutes.

3 Place the liver, bacon and onion in a food processor or blender and add the egg yolks, mixed herbs and rosemary. Blend until all the ingredients are combined and the mixture has a completely smooth consistency.

4 Place the mixture in a dish lined with parchment paper and put in the refrigerator for a couple of hours to set. Serve with vegetable sticks.

SUPERFOOD

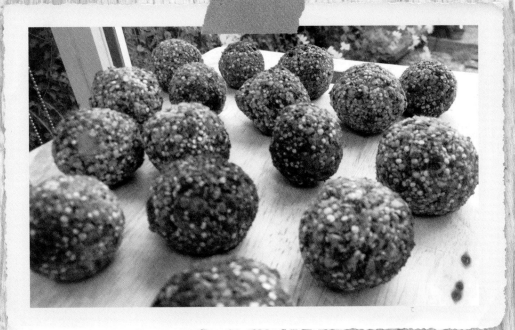

Apricot Energy Shot

Ingredients

★ 4 ounces (100g) quinoa
★ 5 ounces (150g) nuts (we used half cashews and half hazelnuts)
★ 5 ounces (150g) dried unsulphured apricots
★ Juice of 1 lemon
★ 1-½ ounce (40g) hemp or pumpkin seeds
★ 2 tsp maple syrup
★ 1 egg

MAKES:
18 Balls

PREP TIME
15 Minutes

COOKING TIME
15-20 Minutes

1 Preheat the oven to 350°F.

2 Grease a baking tray with a little coconut oil or line with parchment paper.

3 Blend the apricots, egg and lemon juice into a paste.

4 Add the nuts, quinoa and chia seeds and mix into a sticky mixture.

5 Take small handfuls of the mixture and roll into bite-sized balls.

6 Place on the prepared baking tray and bake for 15-20 minutes until golden.

7 Remove from the oven and allow to cool before getting your energy hit.

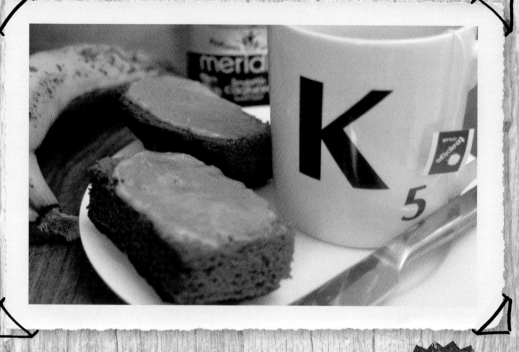

Chocolate Protein Loaf

SERVES: 8

PREP TIME
10 Minutes

COOKING TIME
40-45 Minutes

Ingredients

★ 3 bananas
★ 6 eggs
★ 5 tbsp (80g) vanilla protein powder
★ 2 tbsp chia seeds
★ 1 tbsp ground flaxseed
★ Pinch of nutmeg
★ 1-2 tsp cinnamon
★ 3 tbsp (45g) coconut flour (or ground flaxseed)
★ Pinch of Himalayan Pink or Celtic Sea salt
★ 1 tsp baking powder
★ 1 tsp baking soda
★ ½ tsp Matcha green tea powder (optional)
★ 2 tbsp cocoa powder

1 Preheat the oven to 350°F. Line a loaf pan with parchment paper.

2 Beat the bananas and eggs for 1-2 minutes in a processor or blender.

3 Add the protein powder, chia, flaxseeds, nutmeg, cinnamon, baking soda and salt in a food processor. Sift in the flour, baking powder, cocoa and Matcha powder (if using) and mix again.

4 Pour the batter into the lined tin.

5 Bake for around 40-45 minutes. Before removing from the oven, insert a knife into the middle. When it comes out clean, you know the loaf is baked all the way through.

6 Once baked, remove from the pan and allow to cool. Slice and serve with nut butter or butter.

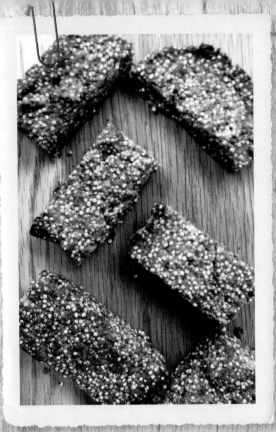

Keen-Wah Energy Bar

Ingredients

★ 5 ounces (150g) quinoa
★ 3.5 ounces (100g) macadamias
★ 5 dates, pitted
★ Juice of half a lemon
★ 3 Tbsp (40g) chia seeds
★ 1 egg
★ Water

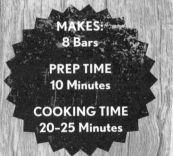

MAKES:
8 Bars

PREP TIME
10 Minutes

COOKING TIME
20–25 Minutes

1 Preheat the oven to 350°F.

2 Grease a baking sheet with a little coconut oil or line with parchment paper.

3 Blend the dates, lemon juice, egg and 1 tablespoon of water into a paste.

4 Add the nuts, quinoa and chia seeds and mix into a sticky mixture.

5 Tip the mixture into the prepared loaf pan and press down firmly with the back of a spoon.

6 Bake in the oven for 20–25 minutes until golden brown.

7 Allow to cool a little before removing from the pan and slicing into bars.

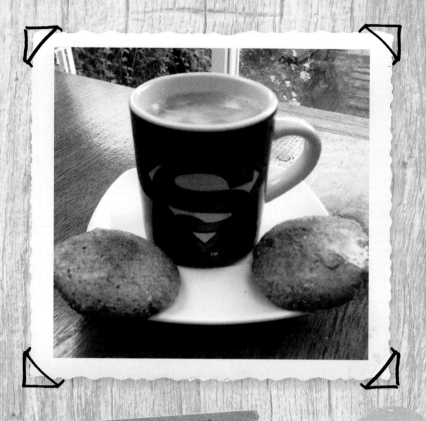

Mini Muscle Cookies

Ingredients

★ 3 tbsp (50g) whey protein
★ 3 tbsp (50g) ground almonds
★ 3-½ tbsp (50ml) almond milk
★ 2 tbsp xylitol or coconut sugar
★ 4 tbsp (60g) almond butter
★ Coconut oil to grease the baking tray

MAKES:
10 Cookies

PREP TIME
10 Minutes

COOKING TIME
10-12 Minutes

1 Preheat the oven to 350°F.

2 In a bowl mix the whey powder, almonds and xylitol.

3 Add in the almond butter and using your hands combine thoroughly with dry ingredients to form a bread crumb-like texture.

4 Add the milk a small amount at a time and combine until the mixture forms a dough. If the mixture becomes too sticky, add some more ground almonds.

5 Grease a baking tray with some coconut oil.

6 Roll the mixture into small balls, place on the baking tray and gently press with the back of a spoon or your thumb into a small cookie shape.

7 Bake in the oven until golden brown.

8 Allow to cool and serve with a double espresso.

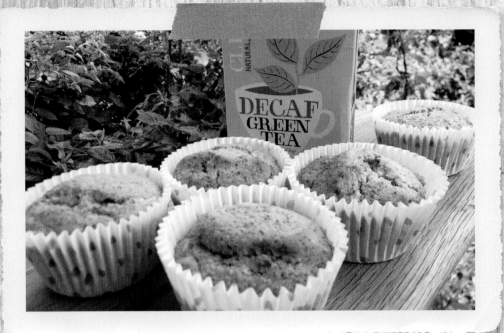

Green Tea Muffins

Ingredients

- ★ 6-½ tbsp (100g) grass fed butter or cashew butter
- ★ 3 tbsp (50g) xylitol or coconut palm sugar
- ★ 5 ounces (150g) ground almonds
- ★ 2 tbsp (30g) tapioca or coconut flour
- ★ 2 green tea bags (fine tea e.g. Clipper)
- ★ 1 tsp baking soda
- ★ 2 eggs, beaten

MAKES:
10 Muffins

PREP TIME
10 Minutes

COOKING TIME
15 Minutes

1 Preheat the oven to 350°F.

2 Line a muffin tray with baking cups.

3 Cream the butter and xylitol in a food processor or bowl.

4 Add the eggs, almonds, flour and baking soda and mix into a cake batter.

5 Rip open the tea bags and pour the tea into the cake mixture. Mix well.

6 Pour the mixture into muffin cases.

7 Bake in the oven for 15-20 minutes until golden brown.

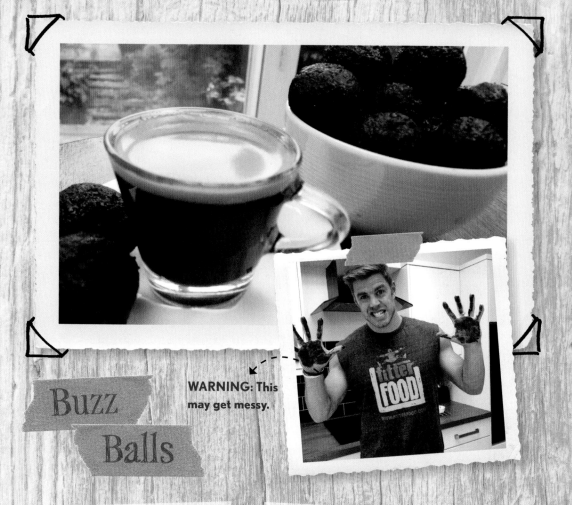

WARNING: This may get messy.

Buzz Balls

Ingredients

★ 4 ounces (100g) 85-90% dark chocolate, melted
★ 4 ounces (100g) macadamias
★ 8 tbsp (100g) desiccated coconut
★ 4 tsp (20g) cocoa powder
★ 3 tbsp (40g) xylitol
★ Shot of espresso (around 80 ml)

MAKES:
22 Balls

PREP TIME
15 Minutes

1 Grease a baking sheet with a little coconut oil.

2 Place the macadamias in a food processor and blend until finely chopped.

3 Place the melted chocolate in a mixing bowl and add the macadamias, coconut, cocoa, xylitol and espresso, and combine thoroughly.

4 The mixture is a little sticky so you can either place teaspoonfuls onto a baking sheet or shape into small balls if you fancy getting a bit messy.

5 Place in the fridge to set for 30 minutes.

Protein Peppermint Thins

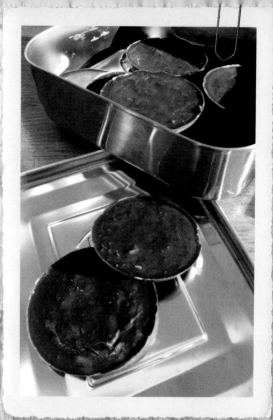

Ingredients

★ 7 tbsp (100g) coconut oil, melted
★ 5 tbsp (80g) vanilla protein powder
★ 1-½ tbsp (20g) desiccated coconut
★ 3 tbsp (50g) cocoa
★ 1 ½ tsp peppermint oil
★ 1 tbsp xylitol
★ 2 tbsp cacoa nibs (optional)

MAKES:
12 Thins

PREP TIME
15 Minutes

1 Grease a muffin pan with coconut oil.

2 Place the coconut oil in a mixing bowl and add the peppermint oil and mix.

3 Stir in the remaining ingredients and combine thoroughly. The mixture should have a liquid consistency so you can easily pour it into the prepared pan.

4 Gently pour a thin layer into the muffin pan to make circular discs.

5 Place in the freezer for 10 minutes to set.

6 Use a butter knife to gently scoop each one out of the tray.

7 Keep refrigerated.

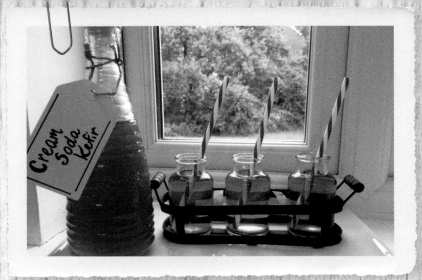

Cream Soda Kefir

This has got to be the easiest way of getting probiotic bacteria into every single member of the household without complaints. Don't be put off by the amount of sugar in this recipe. It plays an essential role in feeding the kefir grains to culture this amazing brew.

1 Boil the water. Place the sugar in the bottom of the Mason jar and dissolve with 2 tsp of boiled water.

2 Allow the remaining water to cool and pour into the Mason jar. Fill it to shoulder level, leaving at least a 1-inch gap at the top to allow for liquid expansion.

3 Place the kefir water grains in the jar of liquid. Place a lid on the jar and fasten tightly.

4 Leave on a kitchen counter for 24 hours to ferment (up to, but no longer than, 48 hours if you prefer a less sweet kefir).

5 Drain the grains from the liquid using a plastic sieve and set the grains aside for your next batch.

6 Add 1 tbsp of vanilla essence to your kefir water, pour into a storage bottle and fasten lid.

7 You can drink immediately but the flavor and fizz improves if you leave for another 24 hours.

8 Store in the fridge and use within 3 days. This allows you just enough time for your next batch to be ready.

9 Burp your bottles every day by opening them to release the build up of gas.

Ingredients

★ 4 tbsp (60g) water kefir grains
★ 4 tbsp (60g) organic brown sugar
★ 1 quart water (ideally distilled/filtered)
★ 1 tbsp vanilla essence

EQUIPMENT

★ 1 liter glass Mason jar or a food grade plastic container.
★ Plastic sieve (it must be plastic).

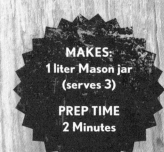

MAKES:
1 liter Mason jar
(serves 3)

PREP TIME
2 Minutes

Speedy Sauerkraut With A Twist

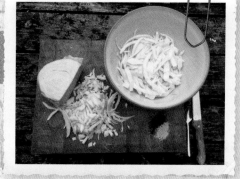

Ingredients

★ 2 pound (1kg) organic white cabbage
★ 2 tbsp fine Himalayan Pink or Celtic Sea salt

"Pimp" your sauerkraut by adding one or a mix of the following, up to 2 teaspoons in total:

★ Toasted caraway seeds
★ Fenugreek seeds
★ Mustard seeds
★ Chopped fresh ginger
★ Turmeric
★ Red pepper flakes
★ Coriander
★ Cumin
★ Whole garlic cloves
★ Bay leaves

Optional topping where needed:
★ 1 tsp fine Himalayan Pink or Celtic Sea salt
★ 1 cup of distilled water

SUPERFOOD

MAKES:
1 liter Mason jar

PREP TIME
30 Minutes

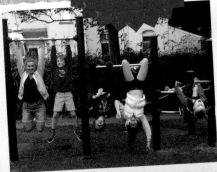

1 Finely chop the cabbage, or use a food processor to save time.

2 Placed chopped cabbage in a large bowl and add the additional ingredients if "pimping" at this stage.

3 Mix in the salt. Rest the ingredients for 30 minutes to allow a natural brine to form from the cabbage.

4 Place everything into the Mason jar, squashing down the ingredients as you go to ensure they are tightly packed in.

5 There should be a layer of brine covering the top of the vegetables. If the vegetables didn't produce enough liquid and the top layer is exposed to air, add some salted water (a mix of 1 tsp salt to 1 cup water) to make sure every strand of cabbage is submerged. Place a lid on the jar, fasten tightly and stand on a saucer in a warm place.

6 Check the cabbage after the second day in case any vegetables are exposed to the air. If so, push them back into the brine.

7 Take a little taste of the sauerkraut each day to check it. Once the salty taste has subsided (this usually takes 5-7 days), it's ready.

8 Store the sauerkraut in the fridge in a container with a fastened lid and use within 2 months.

Claire Harding is a mentor on our Fitter 365 Membership website. She has an autoimmune condition called psoriasis and has been using nutrition and healthy lifestyle habits to rebuild her gut health and regulate her immune system. After experiencing incredible improvements in her symptoms, she embarked on a mission to get the whole family eating fermented foods and developed some super quick and awesome recipes so they became a family favorite.
These are just two of **Claire's Creative Ferments**.

219

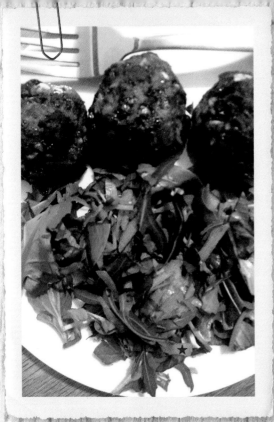

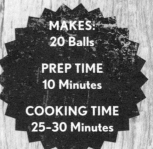

MAKES:
20 Balls

PREP TIME
10 Minutes

COOKING TIME
25–30 Minutes

Crackin' Balls

SUPERFOOD

Ingredients

★ 1-¾ pounds (800g) gluten free
   sausages
★ 1 pound (400g) chicken liver
★ ½ pound (200g) blueberries
★ 4 ounces (100g) toasted hazelnuts
   crushed/finely chopped

1 Preheat the oven to 350°F.

2 Place the liver in a food processor and blend for 2-3 minutes into a paste.

3 Using kitchen scissors, cut and peel the skins off the sausages. Add the meat to the food processor and mix until combined with the liver.

4 Fold in the hazelnuts and blueberries with a spoon and pulse the food processor a few times to mix (but don't purée the fruit).

5 Place a sheet of parchment paper on a baking tray and put spoonfuls of the mixture on the tray. The mixture is sticky so it's easiest to use a spoon and shape into small balls.

6 Bake in the oven for 25-30 minutes. Allow to cool. (We actually prefer these served cold!)

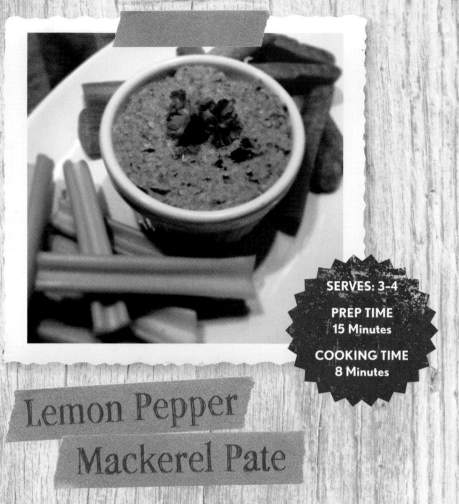

Lemon Pepper
Mackerel Pate

Ingredients

★ 8 ounces (250g) peppered mackerel
  fillets
★ 8 ounces (250g) cremini/baby
  portobello mushrooms
★ ½ white onion, chopped
★ 2 cloves garlic, chopped
★ 3 tbsp fresh lemon juice
★ Handful fresh parsley
★ 1 tbsp olive oil plus more for cooking

Optional

★ ½ cup (150g) butter*
  * This recipe is dairy free but you can
    add butter in as stated in step 4.

1 Saute the onion, garlic and mushrooms in a little olive oil until the onion softens and the mushrooms have browned.

2 Once cooked place all the ingredients into a food processor and blend.

3 Remove the skin from the mackerel and chop into the mushroom mixture. Add the fresh parsley, lemon juice, olive oil and blend all the ingredients thoroughly into a smooth pate.

4 If you prefer a more solid consistency to your pate, add in the butter and blend until smooth. Serve warm or chilled in ramekin dishes with vegetable sticks.

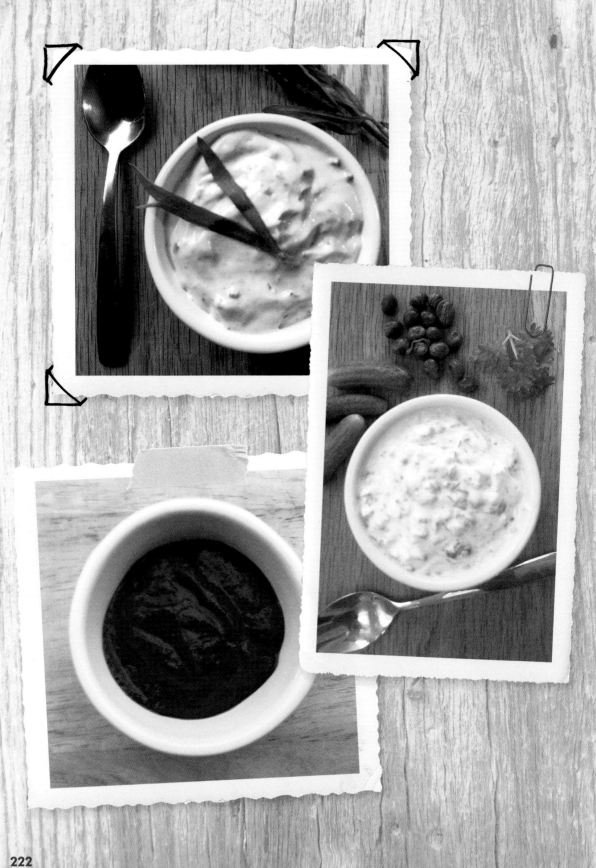

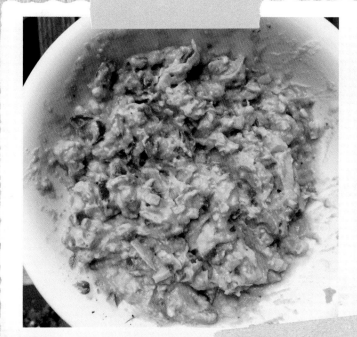

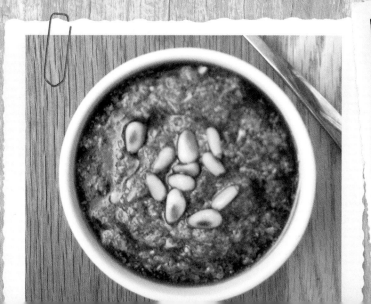

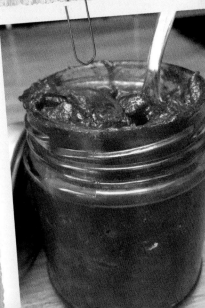

10 Sauces, Dressing & Condiments

Simple
Salad Dressings

Simply place the ingredients in a glass jar with a secure lid and shake, or use a blender/food processor.

Anchovy-Rosemary Vinaigrette
- ★ 2 anchovies, finely chopped
- ★ 3 tbsp apple cider vinegar
- ★ 6 tbsp extra virgin olive oil
- ★ 1 tsp fresh rosemary, chopped
- ★ ¼ tsp Himalayan Pink or Celtic Sea salt
- ★ ⅛ tsp freshly ground black pepper (6 turns on a pepper mill)

Lime and Cumin Dressing
- ★ Juice of 3 limes
- ★ 4 tbsp extra virgin olive oil
- ★ ¼ tsp ground cumin
- ★ ¼ tsp Himalayan Pink or Celtic Sea salt
- ★ ⅛ tsp freshly ground black pepper (6 turns on a pepper mill)

Mustard and Tarragon Vinaigrette
- ★ 4 tsp Dijon mustard
- ★ 2 tbsp apple cider vinegar
- ★ 6 tbsp extra virgin olive oil
- ★ 1 tbsp chopped fresh tarragon
- ★ ¼ tsp Himalayan Pink or Celtic Sea salt
- ★ ⅛ tsp freshly ground black pepper (6 turns on a pepper mill)

Dead Easy Dressing
Grab an empty jam jar (or equivalent). Add any of the three ingredient options below, and **SHAKE**!

- ★ 1 egg yolk, ½ a freshly squeezed lemon and 1 dsp olive oil.
- ★ 2 tsp wholegrain mustard, plus 2 tsp apple cider vinegar. Mix with olive oil to taste.
- ★ 1 tbsp of melted butter or ghee with freshly squeezed lemon juice and 1 tsp capers.

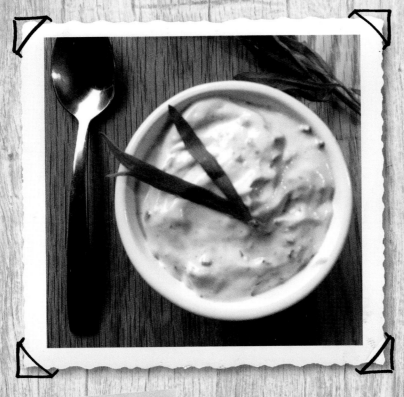

Cheat's Béarnaise Sauce

Ingredients

★ 1 tbsp lemon juice
★ 2 egg yolks
★ 1 tbsp minced shallot
★ ½–1 tsp garlic powder
★ 1-2 tsp Celtic Sea or Himalayan Pink salt
★ Freshly ground black pepper to taste
★ ¾ cup (170g) salted butter
★ 2 tbsp fresh or dried tarragon, minced (add more if you wish)

SERVES: 6

**PREP TIME
5 Minutes**

1 Preheat the oven to 350°F. (or use a microwave).

2 Combine the lemon juice, egg yolks, shallot, garlic powder, salt and pepper in a measuring cup or bowl and blend with a hand blender.

3 Place the butter in a heatproof measuring cup (you ideally need something with a spout) and place it in the oven until the butter has completely melted and is piping hot.

4 Keep the hand blender running while you pour the melted butter into the mixture, moving the blender up and down and from side to side, ensuring you blend all the ingredients. Keep pouring until you have the desired creamy texture.

5 Add the tarragon and blend again until combined thoroughly.

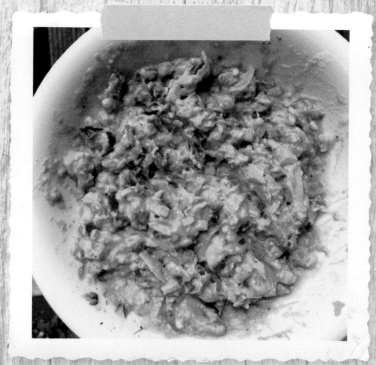

Pimped Guacamole

Ingredients

★ 3 avocados, peeled, stone removed
★ 1 red onion
★ 1 handful of cherry tomatoes, chopped
★ 1 tsp garlic powder
★ 1 handful jalepenos, chopped
★ Juice of 1 lime
★ 2 tbsp Greek yogurt
★ 1 handful fresh cilantro, roughly chopped
★ Celtic Sea or Himalayan Pink salt and freshly ground black pepper
★ ½ tsp cayenne pepper powder (optional)

Place all the ingredients in a large bowl, then mash and mix all the ingredients together. Simples.

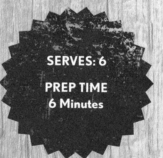

SERVES: 6

PREP TIME
6 Minutes

Tartar Sauce

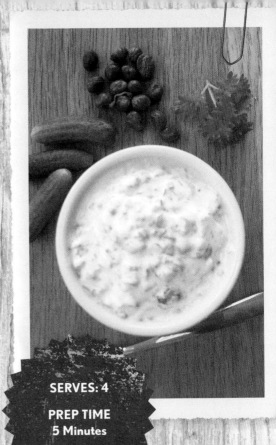

Ingredients

★ 3 heaping tbsp Greek yogurt
  (you can also use sheep's or
  goat's yogurt)
★ 1 heaping tbsp capers, finely chopped
★ 2 tbsp cornichons, finely chopped
★ 1 handful of fresh parsley, chopped
★ Celtic Sea or Himalayan Pink salt

Mix all the ingredients together in a bowl. Taste
and add more seasoning if necessary. **BOSH**

SERVES: 4

**PREP TIME
5 Minutes**

Super Simple Ketchup

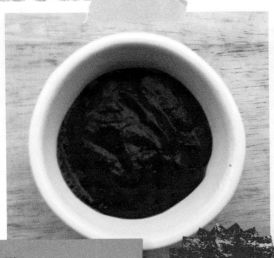

Ingredients

★ ½ cup (100g) tomato purée
★ 2 tbsp balsamic vinegar
★ 6 tbsp water
★ Celtic Sea or Himalayan Pink salt
  and freshly ground black pepper
★ 1 tsp xylitol or raw honey (optional)

SERVES: 4

**PREP TIME
2 Minutes**

TIP

If adding xylitol, you
can grind it into a fine
powder in a coffee grinder
to provide a better ketchup
consistency.

Mix all the ingredients together in a bowl, taste
and add extra sweetener if necessary. **BOSH**

227

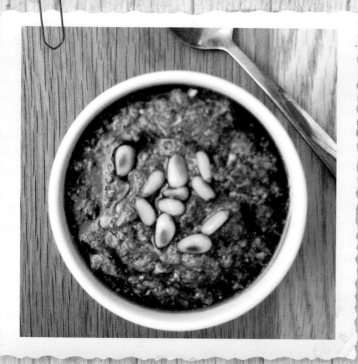

Homemade
Pesto

Ingredients

★ 2 tbsp olive oil
★ A couple of large handfuls fresh basil
★ 1 clove garlic, peeled
★ 2 tbsp Parmesan, finely grated
★ 1 handful pine nuts
★ Celtic Sea or Himalayan Pink salt
  and freshly ground black pepper
★ 1-2 tsp lemon juice

1 Heat a nonstick saucepan on medium heat and cook the pine nuts without any oil for 3-5 minutes. Shake the pan to keep them from burning. Once golden, set aside.

2 Place all the pesto ingredients in a food processor and blend into a thick, creamy consistency. Add more olive oil if required. Blend just enough so the pine nuts are still a little intact to add crunch to the pesto.

SERVES: 2

PREP TIME
5 Minutes

COOKING TIME
**5 Minutes to toast
the pine nuts**

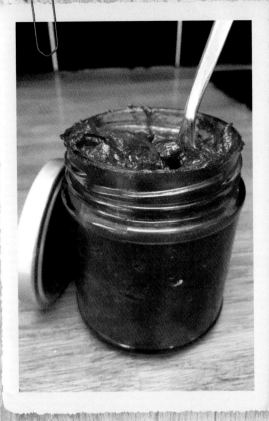

Ingredients

★ 1 tbsp olive oil
★ Half an onion, peeled and finely
  chopped
★ 1 cup (250ml) tomato purée
★ 2 tbsp Worcestershire sauce
★ 2 tbsp xylitol
★ 4 tbsp water
★ ½ tsp garlic powder
★ 1 tbsp apple cider vinegar
★ 1 tsp chili powder
★ Celtic Sea or Himalayan Pink salt
  and freshly ground black pepper

1 Heat the olive oil in a frying pan over medium heat and add the onions to cook for around 12 minutes until soft. Stir occasionally.

2 Mix the remaining ingredients together in a bowl and add to the pan. Simmer for another 15 minutes, stirring occasionally.

3 Leave to cool. Refrigerate and enjoy.

SERVES: 4–6

PREP TIME
5 Minutes

COOKING TIME
30 Minutes

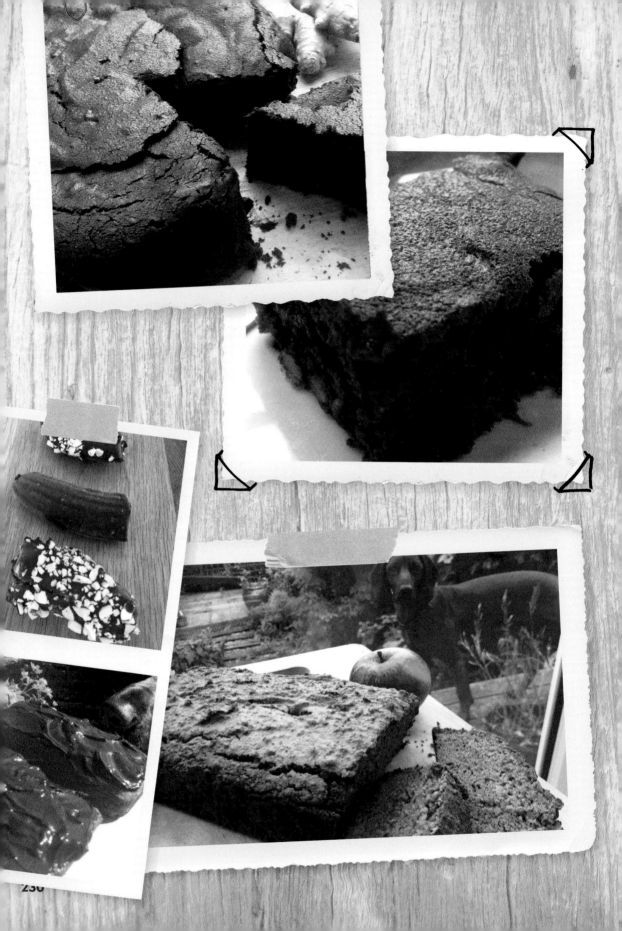

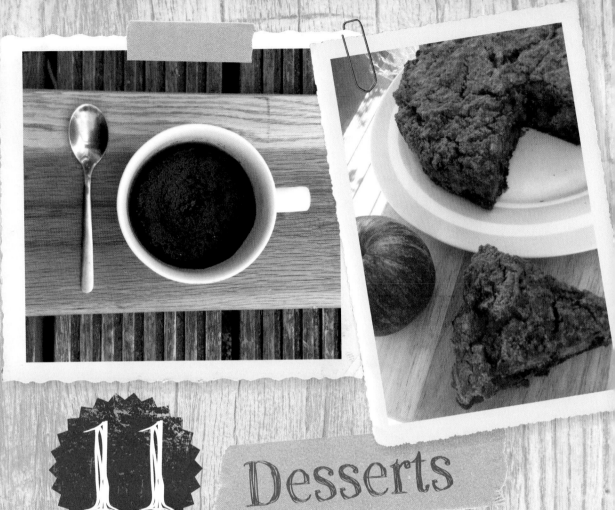

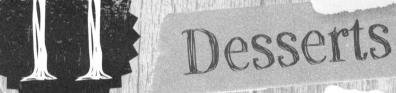

11 Desserts

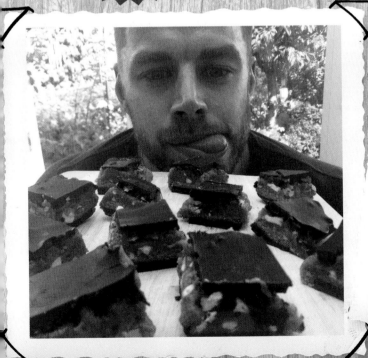

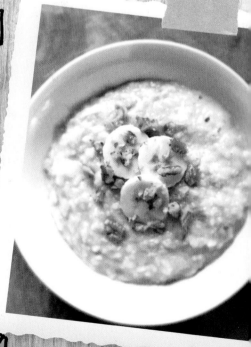

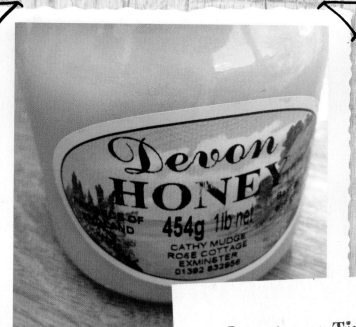

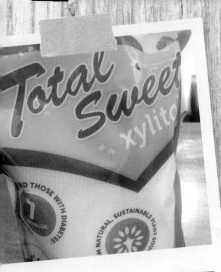

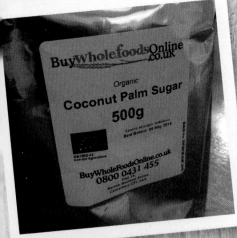

Sweetener Tips

In each recipe we have recommended either honey, xylitol, coconut palm sugar, cane sugar or stevia. In terms of which you choose, this is very much down to personal preference and health goals. If you are significantly overweight, both stevia and xylitol have little impact on blood sugar levels.

Otherwise, honey has fantastic health benefits with antioxidants and enzymes that make it a great natural sweetener. Look for brands with labels like local, organic or cold processed. Unrefined cane sugar or coconut palm sugar are better options if the recipe requires a certain ratio of dry and wet ingredients.

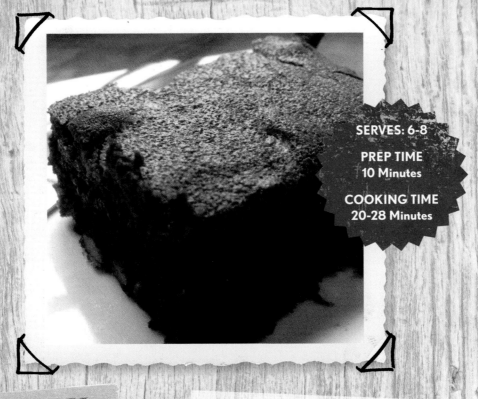

SERVES: 6-8

PREP TIME
10 Minutes

COOKING TIME
20-28 Minutes

BOSH Brownie

Ingredients

★ ½ cup (150g) butter
★ ½ cup (150g) dark chocolate (85% cocao)
★ 3 eggs
★ 1 tsp cinnamon
★ ¾ cup (180g) coconut palm sugar (you can substitute raw honey or xylitol)
★ 7 tbsp (100g) ground almonds
★ ½ – 1 tsp Himalayan Pink or Celtic Sea salt
★ 1 tsp vanilla extract
★ 5 tbsp (80g) pecans, roughly chopped

1 Preheat the oven to 350°F. Line a 9" x 9" brownie pan with parchment paper.

2 Melt the butter and chocolate together in a heat resistant bowl suspended over a saucepan of simmering water.

3 Beat the eggs, coconut sugar, vanilla, cinnamon, ground almonds and salt together in a food processor or using a hand whisk until it forms a cake batter.

4 Once the chocolate and butter have melted, remove from the heat and beat in the egg mixture. Finally, stir in the chopped pecans.

5 Pour the mixture into the prepared pan and bake for around 20-28 minutes. (Ours took 26 minutes!) The top of the brownie should have a light brown crust that is starting to crack. Before removing from the oven, insert a knife/skewer into the middle. It shouldn't wobble but should still be fudgy in the middle. If in doubt, it's better to remove from the oven, check properly and put them back in. It's easy to overcook brownies.

6 Once baked, remove from the oven and allow to cool for 20 minutes before cutting into squares.

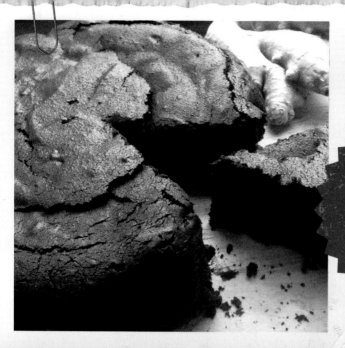

MAKES:
10-12 Slices

PREP TIME
20 Minutes

COOKING TIME
30-40 Minutes (but depends on your oven)

Chocolate Ginger Cake

Ingredients

★ 2 cups (450g) dark chocolate (at least 75% cocao)
★ 8 tbsp unsalted butter
★ 2 tbsp finely grated fresh ginger
★ 2 tsp powdered ginger
★ ½ tsp Celtic Sea or Himalayan Pink salt
★ 8 eggs
★ 8 tbsp (120g) xylitol or coconut palm sugar

1 Preheat the oven to 350°F.

2 Line a 9-inch cake pan with parchment paper and set aside.

3 Melt the chocolate and butter in a heat resistant bowl over a saucepan of water on medium heat until melted and smooth. Remove from the heat and set aside.

4 Meanwhile, beat the eggs, sugar or xylitol, fresh ginger, ginger powder and salt in a food processor for 2-3 minutes.

5 In a large bowl, combine the egg mixture with the melted chocolate. Spoon the batter into the prepared cake pan and sprinkle the top with a pinch of salt.

6 Place in the oven and bake for around 30-40 minutes. Check with a skewer. If it comes out clean, it's ready. Remove from the oven and leave to cool in the pan.

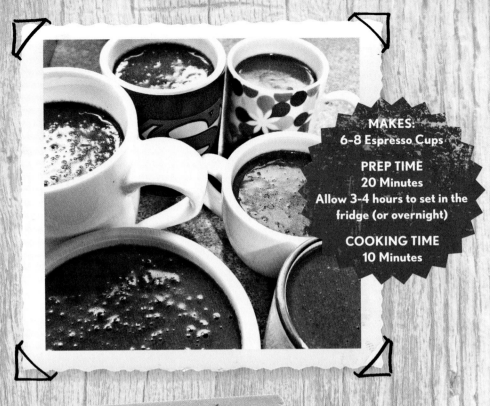

MAKES:
6-8 Espresso Cups

PREP TIME
20 Minutes
Allow 3-4 hours to set in the fridge (or overnight)

COOKING TIME
10 Minutes

Dark Chocolate Delights

Ingredients

★ ½ cup (150g) dark chocolate 85-90% cocao
★ 2 cups (400ml) full fat coconut milk
★ 2-3 tbsp raw honey, maple syrup or Xylitol (*If using xylitol, run through a coffee grinder so the texture is more like icing sugar. This will keep the dessert smooth and creamy.)
★ 1 egg, separated

1 Warm the coconut milk in a pan on low heat. Keep stirring gently and don't allow the milk to boil. After 3-4 minutes, break the chocolate into pieces and add to the milk. Keep stirring to allow the chocolate to melt.

2 Beat the egg white in a blender. Once the chocolate has melted, remove from the heat. Allow to cool for a minute and add the beaten egg white, then stir in the yolk. Combine the ingredients into a smooth ganache.

3 Sweeten to your taste with either honey, maple syrup or xylitol. It's best to taste at this stage to get the sweetness right (plus the mixture is like a thick, hot chocolate). Pour into espresso cups or small dessert dishes and refrigerate for 3-4 hours or overnight.

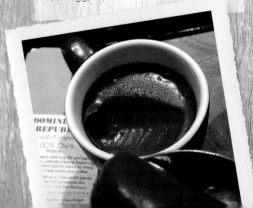

235

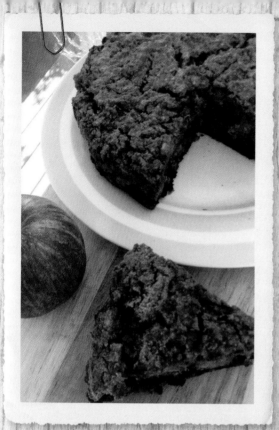

Carrot, Apple and Sultana Cake

Ingredients

★ 3 eggs
★ ¼ cup (60ml) olive oil
★ 1 cups (250g) ground almonds
★ 1 tsp baking soda
★ 1 tsp baking powder
★ 2 tsp cinnamon
★ ½ tsp nutmeg
★ ½ pound (250g) apples (roughly 2 medium apples), cored and grated
★ ½ pound (250g) carrots, grated
★ 4 Tbsp (60g) walnuts, roughly chopped
★ ½ cup (115g) golden raisins

1 Preheat the oven to 325°F.

2 Line an 8-inch cake pan with parchment paper and grease the base and sides with a little butter or olive oil.

3 Beat the eggs and olive oil until smooth.

4 Add the almonds, baking powder and baking soda, cinnamon and nutmeg, and mix again.

5 Finally stir in the apple, carrots, walnuts and raisins.

6 Pour the cake mixture into the prepared cake tin.

7 Bake in the oven for 60-90 minutes. Check the cake after 50 minutes by inserting a clean knife. If the knife comes out dry, the cake is ready.

8 Remove from the oven and allow to cool before slicing and serving.

SERVES: 10

PREP TIME
20 Minutes

COOKING TIME
60-90 Minutes

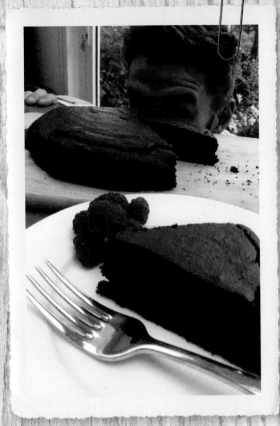

Chocolate Beet Cake

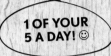

Ingredients

★ 4 eggs
★ 3 Tbsp (35ml) olive oil
★ 7 Tbsp (100g) coconut palm sugar or unrefined cane sugar
★ 9 ounces (250g) cooked beets, chopped
★ 8 Tbsp (120g) ground almonds
★ 1 tsp baking powder
★ ¾ cup (175g) 85% dark chocolate, melted

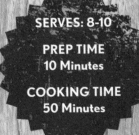

SERVES: 8-10

PREP TIME
10 Minutes

COOKING TIME
50 Minutes

1 Preheat the oven to 350°F.

2 Line an 8-inch cake pan with parchment paper and grease the base and sides with a little butter or olive oil.

3 Beat the eggs, olive oil and sugar in a bowl with a hand whisk or using a food processor until light and fluffy. Add the beets, almonds, baking powder and melted chocolate, and combine thoroughly.

4 Pour the cake mixture into the prepared pan.

5 Bake in the oven for 50 minutes. Check the cake after 40–45 minutes by inserting a clean knife. If the knife comes out dry, the cake is ready.

6 Remove from the oven and allow to cool before slicing.

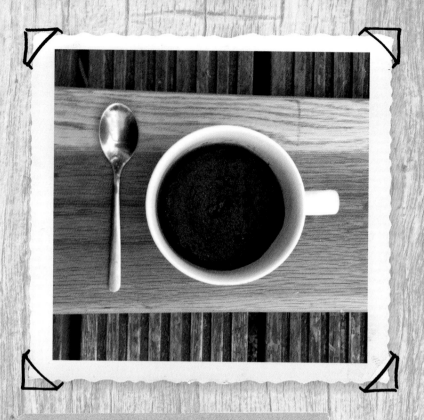

Microwave Molten Mug Cake

Ingredients

★ 1 egg
★ 1 tbsp unsweetened almond milk
★ 1 tbsp xylitol or 2 tsp honey
★ 1 tbsp cocoa
★ 1 tbsp ground almonds
★ ½ tsp orange extract OR peppermint extract
★ 2-3 squares of 85% dark chocolate

1 Place the egg, almond milk and honey or xylitol in a mug and beat with a fork.

2 Add the cocoa, almonds and flavoring of your choice. Combine thoroughly.

3 Drop 2–3 squares of dark chocolate into the mixture and push to the bottom of the mug.

4 Place in the microwave and cook for 1 minute. (Check by popping a knife in the top and checking that it comes out dry). You can also oven cook this for 15 minutes on 350°F.

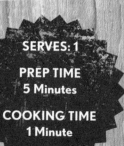

SERVES: 1

PREP TIME
5 Minutes

COOKING TIME
1 Minute

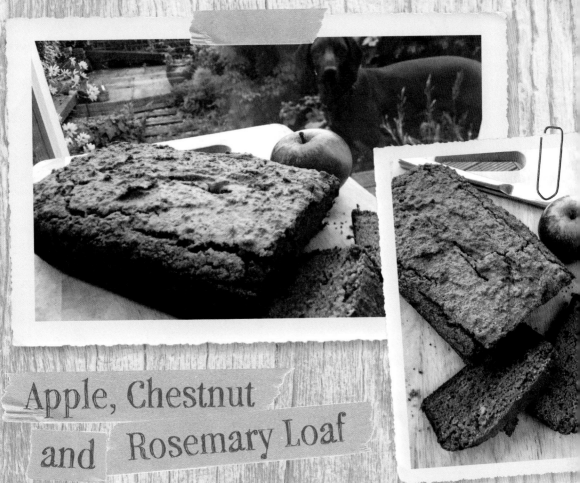

Apple, Chestnut and Rosemary Loaf

Ingredients

★ 3 eggs
★ 4 tbsp (60ml) olive oil
★ Juice of half a lemon
★ ¾ cup (200g) chestnut flour
★ 1 tsp baking soda
★ ½ tsp baking powder
★ 3 tbsp (50g) ground almonds
★ 1 tsp cinnamon
★ Pinch of nutmeg
★ 1 sprig fresh rosemary, finely chopped
★ 3 small apples, cored and grated

SERVES: 8-10

PREP TIME
15 Minutes

COOKING TIME
40-45 Minutes

1 Preheat the oven to 350°F.

2 Line an 8-inch loaf pan with parchment paper and grease the base and sides with a little butter or olive oil.

3 Beat the eggs, olive oil and lemon juice in a bowl or using a food processor until light and fluffy. Add the chestnut flour, almonds, baking powder, baking soda, cinnamon and nutmeg, and mix again.

4 Finally, stir in the grated apple and pour the cake mixture into the prepared loaf pan.

5 Bake in the oven for 40–45 minutes. Check the cake after 35 minutes by inserting a clean knife. If the knife comes out dry, the cake is ready.

6 Remove from the oven and allow to cool before slicing and serving with a little butter.

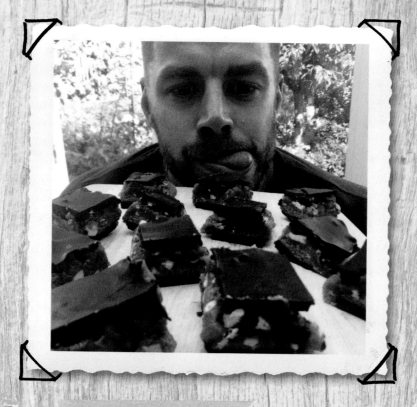

S'nickers in a Twist

Ingredients

★ 11 ounces (300g) dark chocolate (have some extra in case you need to fill gaps)
★ Small handful cashews

FOR THE NOUGAT

★ 1 cup (240g) smooth almond butter
★ 3-4 tbsp coconut flour
★ 4 tbsp coconut palm sugar or xylitol

FOR THE CARAMEL

★ ½ cup (130g) medjool dates
★ 3 tbsp cashew butter
★ 2 tbsp (30g) coconut oil
★ Pinch Celtic Sea or Himalayan Pink salt
★ 4 tbsp water

1 Melt half of the chocolate (5-½ oz/150g) in a glass bowl over simmering water or in a microwave.

2 Line a square pan with parchment paper and pour in the melted chocolate. Place in the freezer to allow to set.

3 Preheat the oven to 350°F.

4 Place the cashews on a baking tray and put in the oven for 10-15 minutes to lightly toast. Keep an eye on them and remove once they begin to turn golden. Set aside to cool.

5 To make the nougat, place the almond butter, coconut flour and palm sugar (or xylitol) in a food processor and blend. The mixture should be solid and sticky like cookie dough. If it's too dry, add a little water or nut butter. If it's too soggy, add a little more coconut flour.

6 Set the nougat aside.

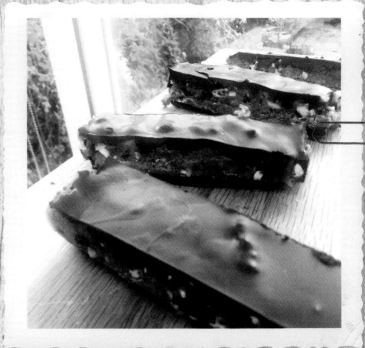

MAKES:
8-10 Small Slices

PREP TIME
30 Minutes
(couple of hours to set)

COOKING TIME
10-15 Minutes

7 To make the caramel, blend the dates into a paste in a food processor. Add the cashew butter, coconut oil, a sprinkle of salt, and blend. To make the caramel consistency, you need to carefully add water little by little. Start with 1 tablespoon and keep the food processor going. Usually 3-4 will turn the mixture into a soft, sticky caramel texture. You can add a little more cashew butter if necessary to make it a little smoother.

8 Crush the toasted cashews into tiny pieces. It's easiest to use your hands for this.

9 Melt your second batch of chocolate (5-½ oz/150g) and set aside.

10 Remove the first batch of chocolate from the freezer and check that it's completely set. Using a spoon or knife, spread a layer of nougat evenly on top of the chocolate.

11 Follow this with a thick layer of caramel and sprinkle over the toasted cashews.

12 Finally, pour over the second batch of melted chocolate and use a knife to spread it evenly over the caramel layer.

13 Place in the fridge for a couple of hours to set. Once set, remove from the pan, peel off the parchment paper and carefully slice into squares.

NOTE

We stuck these in the freezer to stop us eating them and invented S'nickers in a Twist ice cream... nom nom!

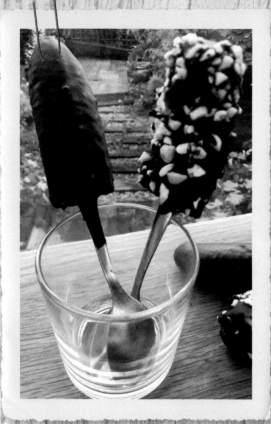

MAKES: 6

PREP TIME
15 Minutes
(Plus 2-3 to freeze)

Banana Choc Ices

Ingredients
★ 3 bananas
★ 3-1/2 ounces (100g) dark chocolate
★ Handful of nuts, crushed

1 Melt the chocolate over a pan of simmering water or in the microwave. Place in wide bowl to make it easy to dip the bananas. Allow the chocolate to cool for 5 minutes so it begins to thicken and is easier to coat the bananas.

2 Place the crushed nuts on a plate.

3 Clear some space in the freezer as you need to work quickly.

4 Slice the bananas in half and insert a teaspoon into each one. Have a glass ready and place it on a tray. (The chocolate will drip a little.)

5 Dip the banana in the chocolate, coat thoroughly and roll in the nuts. Gently place in the glass. (The tray will catch any dripping chocolate.) Work quickly to coat the remaining bananas. (You can begin to place them in the freezer to stop them dripping). Place in the freezer for 5-10 minutes until the chocolate sets.

TIP
If you can get hold of wooden popsicle sticks, you can make your own Banana Feast Bars! Or if you want to save some hassle and aren't too bothered about presentation, you can dip the banana in the chocolate and nuts and simply lay it on the parchment paper.

242

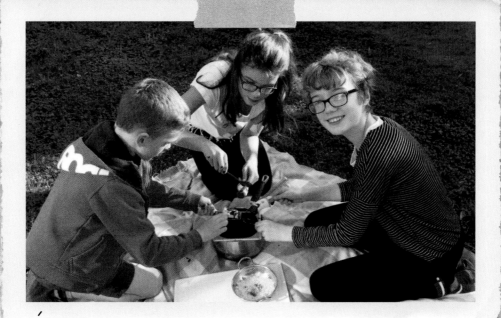

We asked Fitter Food mom Claire Harding to test out the banana choc ices with her family, and they certainly got the thumbs up! This is a great recipe for kids to get into.

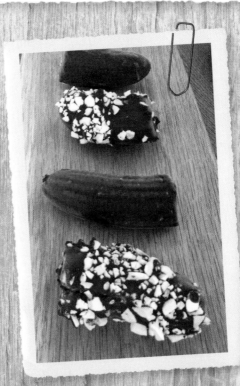

6 Remove from the freezer and gently pull out the teaspoon from each choc ice. Place back in the freezer to set for 2-3 hours or overnight.

7 When serving, wrap a little foil or parchment paper around the choc ice. The chocolate will melt quickly.

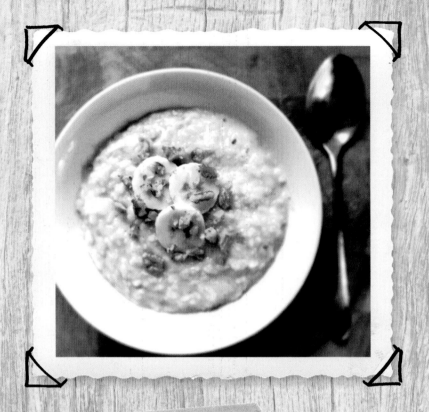

Post Workout
Rice Pudding

Ingredients

★ ¾ cup (200g) cooked rice, cold
  (you can use basmati, white or brown)
★ ½ can coconut milk (shake can well)
★ 1 tbsp butter
★ 1 banana
★ 1-2 tbsp raw honey or xylitol
★ ½ tsp cinnamon
★ 1 tbsp crushed walnuts

OPTIONAL
★ Seeds or berries

1 Add the rice, coconut milk and butter to a saucepan on a low to medium heat and mix through until the mixture starts to thicken.

2 Now mash half the banana and add to the saucepan with the cinnamon and honey, and stir again.

3 Simmer for a few minutes until nice and creamy.

4 Place in bowls and top with the remaining banana (sliced), the cinnamon and crushed walnuts.

SERVES: 2

PREP TIME
3 Minutes

COOKING TIME
5 Minutes

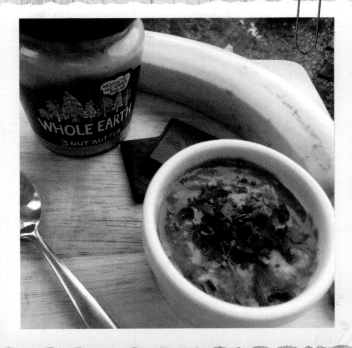

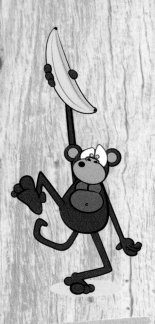

Funky Monkey Pudding

Ingredients
★ 1 frozen banana
★ 1 tbsp chunky nut butter
★ 1 heaping tsp cocoa

Blend the banana into a purée and stir in the nut butter and cocoa.

OPTIONAL
To add a protein hit, stir in a spoonful of chocolate or vanilla protein powder. (Add a little almond milk if necessary.)

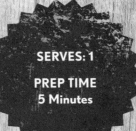

SERVES: 1

PREP TIME
5 Minutes

245

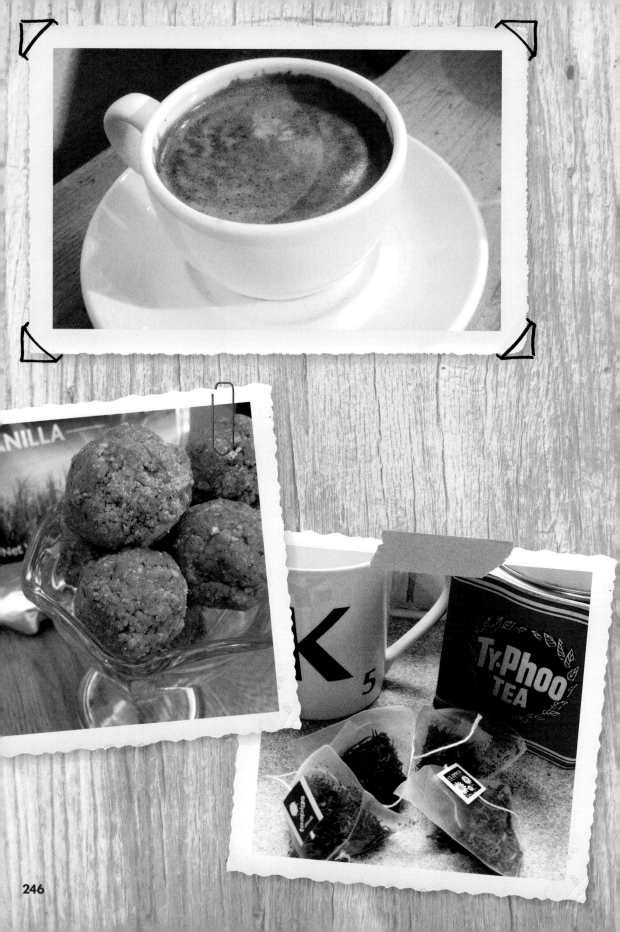

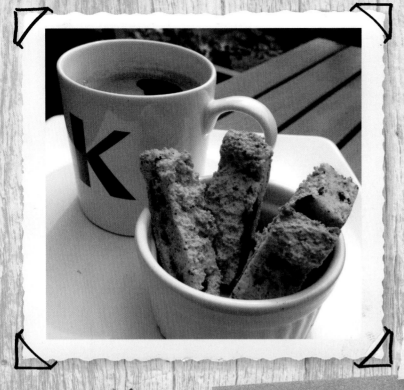

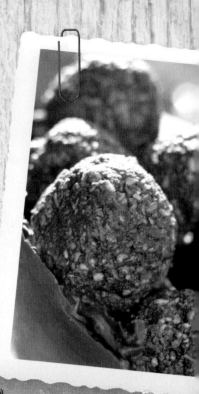

12

After Dinner Bites

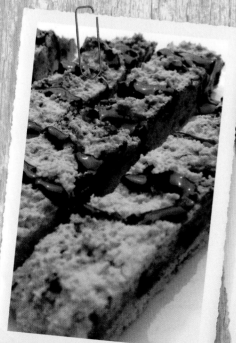

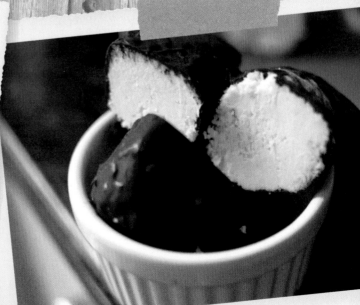

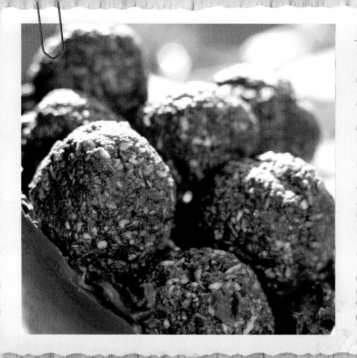

Aprichoc Balls

Ingredients

★ 7 ounces (200g) dark chocolate (85%-90%)
★ 7 ounces (200g) desiccated coconut
★ 9 ounces (250g) unsulphured apricots

MAKES:
22-24 Balls

PREP TIME
15 Minutes
(couple of hours to set)

1 Break the chocolate into small pieces and gently melt in a glass bowl over simmering water. Allow to cool slightly.

2 Place the apricots in a food processor with 2-3 tablespoons of water and blend into a sticky paste. Add the coconut and melted chocolate and mix thoroughly. The mixture should be sticky (so it's easy to roll into balls). If not, add a little more water and mix again.

3 Take handfuls of the mixture and roll into small balls.

4 Place on a baking sheet covered in parchment paper and refrigerate until set.

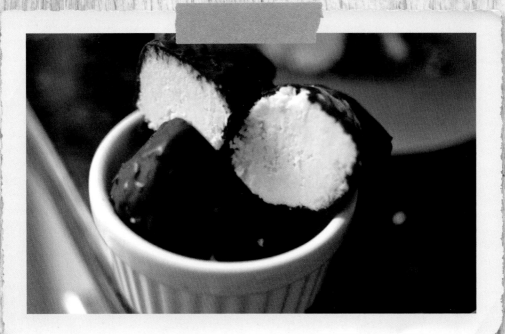

Bounty Bites

Ingredients

★ 6 ounces (160g) desiccated coconut
★ 5 tbsp (80g) coconut cream
★ 4 tsp xylitol or honey
★ 5 ounces (150g) dark chocolate
   (minimum 75% cocao)

MAKES:
8 Balls

PREP TIME
10 Minutes

COOKING TIME
2-3 Hours

1 Place the coconut, coconut cream and sweetener in a bowl and mix together. The mixture should easily stick together; if required add more coconut cream.

2 Gently shape into small bite-sized balls and place on a sheet of parchment paper.

3 Place in the freezer for 2-3 hours until frozen.

4 Once the balls are frozen solid, melt the chocolate in a heat resistant bowl over a saucepan of simmering water.

5 Remove the coconut balls from the freezer and dip each one into the melted chocolate. Roll it around to ensure it is completely coated in chocolate.

6 Arrange the chocolate-coated coconut balls on a baking sheet covered with greaseproof paper and place in the fridge to set.

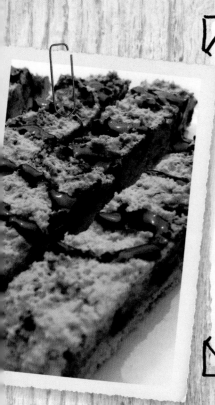

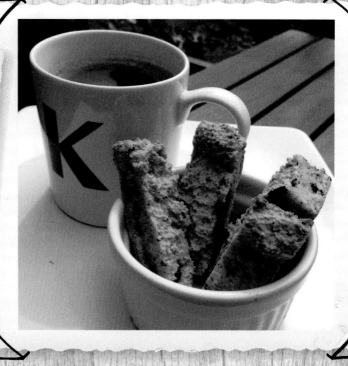

BOSH Biscotti

Ingredients

★ 4 eggs, beaten
★ 5 tbsp (75ml) coconut oil, melted
★ 6 heaping tbsp honey
★ ½ tsp vanilla extract
★ ½ tsp almond extract
★ 1-½ cups (350g) ground almonds
★ 3 tbsp coconut flour
★ ½ tsp baking soda
★ 2 ounces (50g) dark chocolate,
   85% cocao, chopped

MAKES:
10-12 Large Biscotti

PREP TIME
15 Minutes

COOKING TIME
45 Minutes

1 Preheat the oven to 350°F.
Grease a large baking tray with a little butter.

2 In a large bowl, whisk together the beaten eggs, coconut oil, honey, vanilla and almond extract.

3 Add the ground almonds, coconut flour and baking soda, and stir in thoroughly. Mix in the chocolate chunks.

4 Spread the batter out on the baking tray until about an inch thick before placing in the oven to cook for 25-30 minutes. (Cooking time depends on the oven, so keep an eye on it.)

5 Once the batter has turned golden brown, remove from the oven and cut into ½ inch pieces. Lay each slice on its side on the baking sheet, spread them out evenly and place back in the oven for 10 minutes before flipping them over. Turn the oven down slightly to about 325°F.

6 Once golden, remove from the oven and allow to cool before munching.

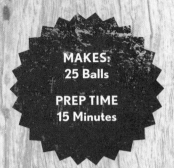

MAKES:
25 Balls

PREP TIME
15 Minutes

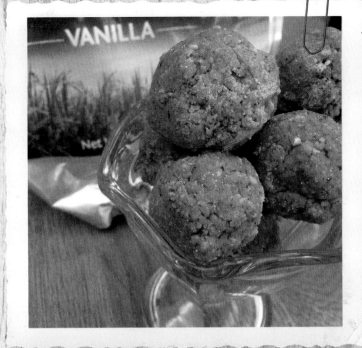

Goji Protein Truffles

Ingredients

- ★ ¾ cup (200g) mixed nuts and coconut flakes
- ★ 2 tbsp goji berries
- ★ 4 tbsp (50g) coconut flour
- ★ 7 tbsp (100g) vanilla protein powder
- ★ Generous sprinkle of Himalayan Pink or Celtic Sea salt
- ★ 1 heaping tsp cinnamon
- ★ 1 tsp vanilla extract
- ★ 3 tbsp (50g) coconut oil
- ★ 5 tbsp (70g) cashew butter
- ★ 2-3 tbsp water

OPTIONAL

If the protein powder isn't sweetened you may wish to add some raw honey, liquid stevia or xylitol to taste.

1 Place the nuts, coconut and goji berries in a food processor and blend until finely chopped.

2 Add the flour, protein powder, cinnamon and salt.

3 Finally blend in the coconut oil, cashew butter and vanilla extract.

4 The mixture should start to form a sticky dough. Add a tablespoonful of water to help it bind. You should be able to take a small handful and shape into a small ball. (Squeeze it to help the mixture bind.) If the mixture is still falling apart, add another 1-2 tablespoonfuls of water and try again.

5 Place the balls in the fridge to set.

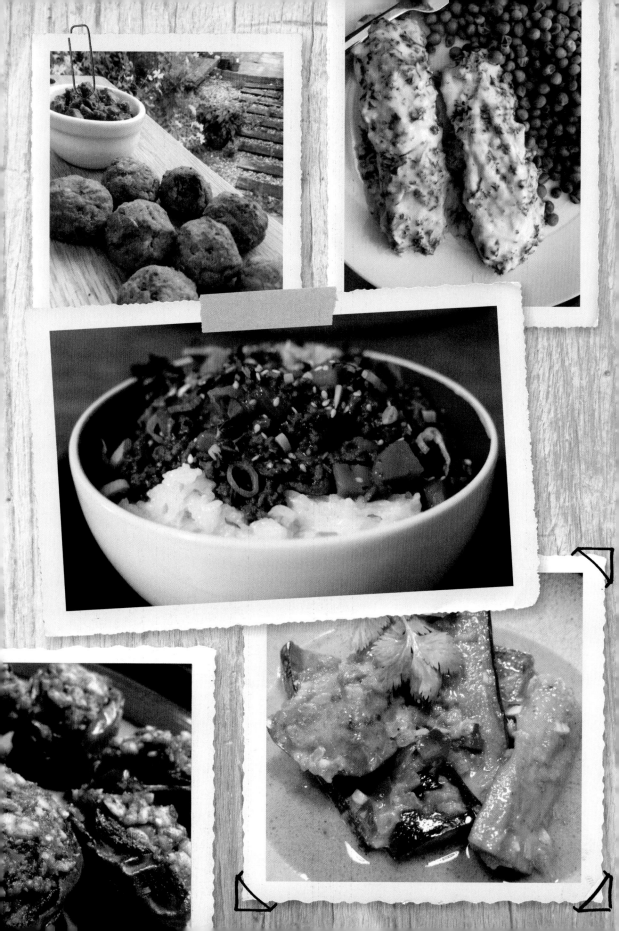

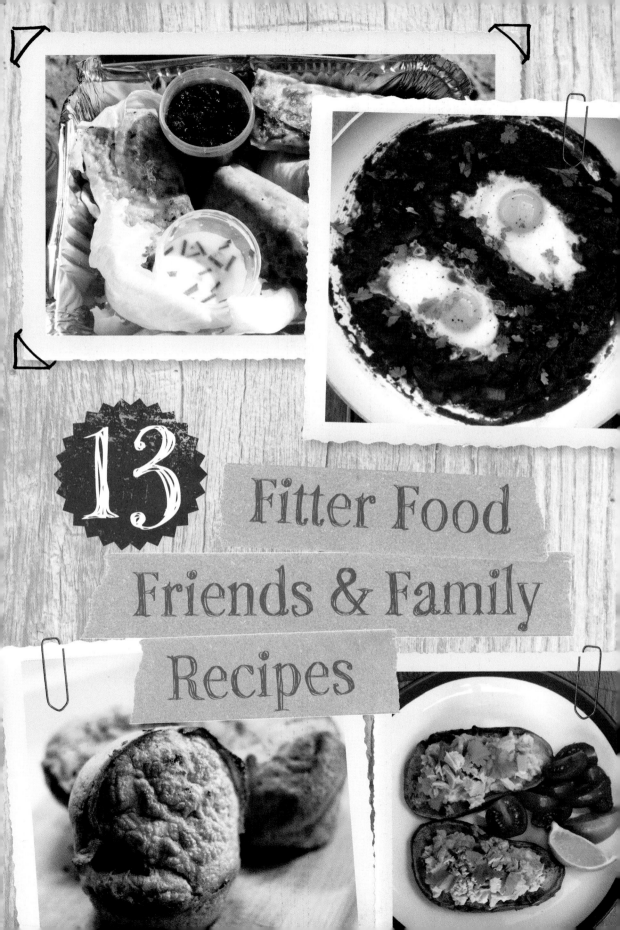

13
Fitter Food
Friends & Family
Recipes

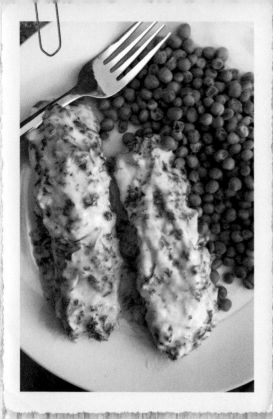

Dad's Leek, Parsley and Potato Salmon

Ingredients

- ★ 2 tbsp coconut oil or butter
- ★ 3 garlic cloves peeled and finely chopped
- ★ 1 leek, finely chopped
- ★ ¾ pound (375g) white potatoes, chopped
- ★ 1-¾ cup (400ml) chicken stock
- ★ ¾ cup (150-200ml) cream
- ★ Large handful fresh parsley, finely chopped
- ★ 4 salmon fillets

1 Heat the coconut oil in a saucepan on medium heat before adding the garlic, leek and potatoes and cooking for around 5 minutes, stirring occasionally.

2 Preheat the oven to 350°F.

3 Add the chicken stock to the saucepan with the potatoes and leeks, stir well, bring to a boil and cook for around 15 minutes or until the potatoes are soft.

4 Add the cream and then use a hand blender or food processor to blend all the ingredients into a smooth sauce. Make sure there are no lumps remaining. Stir in the parsley.

5 Place the salmon fillets into a baking dish and pour over the sauce, ensuring each fillet is fully coated. Keep any leftover sauce for other dishes—it's the best!

6 Place in the oven to cook for 20-25 minutes.

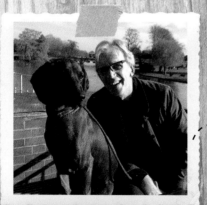

"This recipe is dedicated to my sister Christine. It was one of the last meals I cooked for her before she lost her battle with cancer. I have fond memories of our last moments together, sharing delicious food and laughter." CHRIS MARSDEN

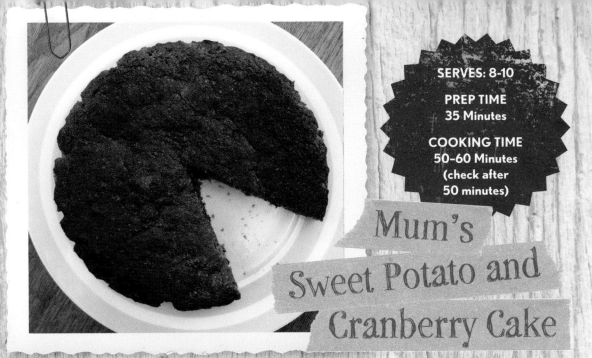

SERVES: 8-10

PREP TIME
35 Minutes

COOKING TIME
50-60 Minutes
(check after
50 minutes)

Mum's Sweet Potato and Cranberry Cake

Ingredients

★ ¾ cup (200g) ground almonds
★ 1½ tsp baking soda
★ 4 eggs
★ 5 tbsp (75g) butter
★ 200g xylitol
★ ¾ cup (200g) sweet potato, cooked & peeled
★ ⅓ cup (75g) walnuts, chopped
★ ½ cup (100g) dried cranberries

1 Line a 9-inch cake pan with parchment paper and grease with butter.

2 Preheat the oven to 350°F.

3 Place the sweet potato, almonds, baking soda and butter in a bowl and mash together. Stir in the walnuts and cranberries.

4 In a separate bowl, whisk together the eggs and xylitol until light and fluffy.

5 Fold the eggs into the potato mixture and combine thoroughly.

6 Pour into the prepared pan and bake for around 40-50 minutes. Check the cake after 40 minutes by inserting a clean knife. If the knife comes out dry, the cake is ready.

7 Remove from the oven and allow to cool before slicing and serving.

"I'm always looking for creative cake recipes with different combinations of fruits, nuts, vegetables and spices that mean you can cut back on the sugar. We spend our summers in Portugal, and the Portuguese often use sweet potatoes in cakes, pies and even ice cream, so I thought I'd give it a go. This one worked a treat!" CELINE MARSDEN

Meg and Tom's Paleo Yorkshire Puddings

TIP
If your oven is too hot, the puddings will burn, so it's best to start with a higher temperature and gradually reduce so the puddings brown but don't burn.

Ingredients

★ 4 eggs
★ ¾ cup (200g) tapioca flour
★ ¾ cup (200ml) almond milk)
★ ¼ tsp baking soda
★ Olive oil, butter or coconut oil for greasing the tray

MAKES:
6 Yorkshire Puddings

PREP TIME
15 Minutes

COOKING TIME
20-22 Minutes

1 Preheat the oven to 425°F.

2 Crack the eggs into a measuring cup and make a note of the fluid level. Place the eggs in a blender. Add milk to the blender to the same level that the eggs reached when measured in the cup.

3 Now measure the same amount of flour (dry the measuring cup first so the flour doesn't stick) and add to the blender. Finally, add the baking soda and blend into a smooth batter.

4 Place ½ teaspoon of oil into each muffin cup in the tin. Heat the muffin tray on a stove until the oil is smoking. You can do this in a hot oven but for best results use the stove. Pour the mixture into each muffin cup, filling up to ¾ full. Place in the oven for 12 minutes until risen, then reduce the temperature to 400°F and cook for another 10 minutes.

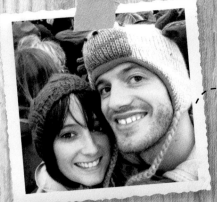

"We love following Fitter Food principles daily, but Meg is particularly proud of her Yorkshire roots and found herself missing that northern Sunday staple: the Yorkshire Pudding. So we came up with this gem of a recipe." TOM AND MEG (KERIS'S BROTHER AND HIS GIRLFRIEND)

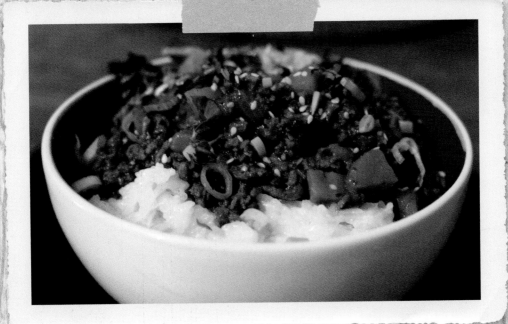

Meg and Tom's Bangin' Beef Bulgogi

Ingredients

★ 1 pound (500g) ground beef or lamb
★ 2 slices bacon, diced (optional)
★ 2 tbsp xylitol
★ 3 tbsp tamari
★ 1 tbsp sesame oil
★ 1 tsp crushed red pepper flakes
★ ½ tsp ground ginger
★ 3 cloves garlic, crushed
★ 1 large onion, finely chopped
★ 1 carrot, diced
★ Half a savoy cabbage, shredded

SERVES: 2-4

PREP TIME
15 Minutes

COOKING TIME
20 Minutes

This Korean-inspired dish is something we have when we fancy something different from the usual burgers, bolognese or chili.

1 Heat the sesame oil in a pan, add the garlic and fry for one minute. Add the onion and carrot and cook until soft. Set the vegetables to one side.

2 Fry the meat and bacon until brown and drain off any excess fat. Add the vegetables back into the pan.

3 In a bowl, mix 2-3 tablespoons of boiling water with the xylitol and stir until it dissolves. Add the tamari, sesame oil, pepper flakes and ginger, and mix. Add to the meat and vegetables in the pan and simmer for 5 minutes.

5 Season to taste and serve with coconut rice (page 189) and steamed savoy cabbage.

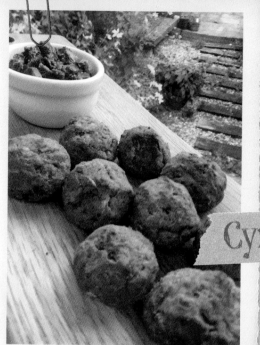

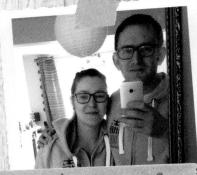

Cynneth and Kerry's Lil' Balls Of Greatness

Ingredients

★ 1 medium sweet potato, peeled and cut in half
★ 1 large egg
★ ¼ cup of coconut or almond flour
★ 1 heaping tsp smoked paprika
★ 1 heaping tsp garlic powder
★ ½ tsp Himalayan Pink or Celtic Sea salt
★ Olive oil for cooking (if using Method 1)

MAKES:
12–15 Balls

PREP TIME
15 Minutes

COOKING TIME
3–5 minutes frying or
15–20 minutes baking

1 Boil the sweet potato for 3–5 minutes.
NOTE It shouldn't be too soft, as it needs to be grated. Rinse in cold water and allow to cool.

2 Beat the egg in a bowl. In a separate bowl, mix the dry ingredients together. Grate the sweet potato into the beaten egg and mix. It's easiest to mix little-by-little so that you don't mash the sweet potato too much.

3 Add the dry ingredients into the egg and grated sweet potato. Once everything is all mixed up, roll into small balls (of greatness) around 1 inch in diameter. There are two ways they can be cooked:

METHOD 1—FRYING

Heat a generous amount of olive oil in a pan and place the balls in the oil. They do burn quickly, so they will need to be turned a lot. They can fall apart sometimes too, so care needs to be taken when turning them. Using a tablespoon works well. Keep turning until they are crispy and brown on the outside (around 3–5 minutes).

METHOD 2—BAKING

Preheat the oven to 400°F.
Place the balls on a baking tray lined with parchment paper. Bake for 15–20 minutes.

"We met Keris and Matt in our shop and were intrigued with Fitter Food. We started one of their plans in March 2015 and haven't looked back since. We are both healthier, happier, more energized, have lost weight and never felt better! We really enjoy cooking (and eating!), and the variety of dishes that Matt and Keris share have opened up a whole new world of eating awesome food. Their recipes are easy, tasty and healthy! Being a part of the Fitter Food family has been a great journey and is now a huge part of our lives. We can't ever see that changing!" CYNNETH AND KERRY BONANOS

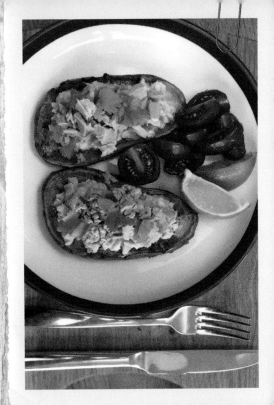

Sweet Potato Toast

Ingredients

★ 2 large sweet potatoes
★ 1 tsp paprika
★ 1 tsp dried rosemary
★ 1 tbsp coconut oil or olive oil for cooking

TOPPING

★ 1 avocado
★ Juice of 1 lime
★ 1 tbsp olive oil
★ Celtic Sea or Himalayan Pink salt and freshly ground black pepper
★ 1 can tuna
★ Handful of cherry tomatoes
★ Handful of spinach

SERVES:
6–8 Slices of Toast

PREP TIME
10 Minutes

COOKING TIME
30-35 Minutes

We came up with this recipe after a crazy, stressful week where we had been working late most evenings. We were just too tired to cook and couldn't face spending too long in the kitchen. I'd seen a picture of potato toast on Instagram so decided to have a go. This is the perfect quick meal for those extra-long working days. We've also had it topped with eggs for breakfast.

1 Preheat the oven to 350°F.

2 Slice a sweet potato lengthways into slices around ⅓-inch thick. Sprinkle with the paprika and rosemary (or use any of your favorite herbs). Place on a baking sheet and spoon over some coconut oil or drizzle over olive oil. Allow to cook for 30-35 minutes.

3 Make a quick guacamole by mashing the avocado with lime juice, olive oil and seasoning.

4 Once the sweet potato slices are cooked to your liking, remove from the oven and top with the guacamole, tuna, tomatoes and spinach.

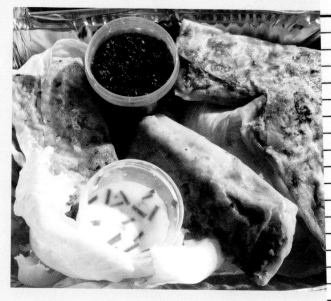

Kefir Garlic and Chive Dip

A great simple way to get some probiotics into you.

1 tsp raw honey
2-½ ounces kefir (ferment for a slightly longer period if needed to thicken)
1 handful chopped chives
2 cloves garlic
Celtic Sea or Himalayan Pink salt and freshly ground black pepper

Mix together the honey, kefir and garlic. Add the chives and seasoning. Serve chilled with some "Big Dippers."

SERVES: 4
PREP TIME 5 Minutes

Fitter Food Mom Claire Harding's
Big Dippers

Ingredients

★ 3 tbsp (50g) butter (ghee or coconut oil can be substituted)
★ 1 pound (500g) ground lamb
★ 2 medium sweet potatoes, peeled, steamed and mashed
★ 1 large onion, finely chopped
★ 6 cloves garlic
★ 1 handful fresh rosemary
★ 1 handful fresh thyme
★ 1 tbsp turmeric
★ 1 pinch of Celtic Sea or Himalayan Pink salt and freshly ground black pepper
★ 1 packet spring roll wrappers

MAKES: 16

PREP TIME
10 Minutes

COOKING TIME
30–40 Minutes

This is one of our favorite family recipes that gives everyone a thrill! The bonus with these is that the kids absolutely love making them, and they're perfect as party food or to pop in to a school lunch.

1 Melt the butter in a frying pan and brown the onions, garlic and ground lamb. Add the herbs, salt and pepper. Mix in the sweet potato, then set aside to cool.

2 Once cooled, place 2 teaspoons of the mixture into the spring roll wrapper and seal into a long sausage shape. (Fold from the bottom first, then both sides, rolling up to the top.)

3 Place sealed edge down onto a baking tray and bake in an oven at 400°F until brown and crispy.

4 Serve with kefir, chive and garlic dip and tarty tomato relish... and enjoy!

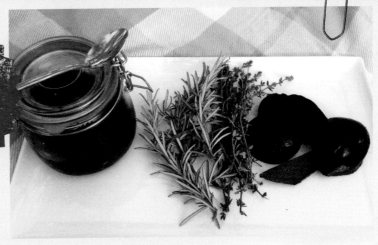

MAKES: 17 oz
(enough to serve 8)

PREP TIME
10 Minutes

COOKING TIME
30-40 Minutes

Tarty
Nomato Relish

Ingredients

★ 1 tsp butter (ghee or coconut oil can be substituted)
★ 2 medium sized beets, chopped
★ 1 gem squash
★ 1 large onion, finely chopped
★ 2 carrots, chopped
★ 5 cloves garlic
★ 1 handful fresh rosemary
★ 1 handful fresh thyme
★ ½ tsp dried basil
★ ½ tsp oregano
★ ½ tsp sage
★ ¾ cup (200ml) water
★ 1-¾ tbsp (25ml) balsamic vinegar
★ 1-¾ tbsp (25ml) apple cider vinegar
★ Juice of 1 lemon
★ Celtic Sea or Himalayan Pink salt and freshly ground black pepper

I have to follow an autoimmune diet which eliminates nightshades, and gosh do I miss tomatoes! This is an alternative to a tangy tomato relish. Discovering this was life changing and made the lack of nightshades in my nutrition much more bearable.

1 Steam the beets, squash and carrots until soft. Fry the onion and garlic in some butter or ghee until soft and slightly browned.

2 In a separate bowl, blend together the vinegars, water and lemon juice. Place the vegetables, onion, garlic and vinegar mixture in a food processor or blender and blend.

3 Pour into a saucepan, add in the herbs and seasoning and simmer for around 20 minutes or until the liquid has reduced down.

4 Serve chilled with some "Big Dippers" and enjoy.

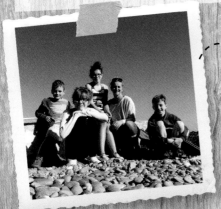

"I'm part of the Fitter Food team and mentor their online programs. I follow an autoimmune diet, so many of my recipes include fermented foods and eliminate nightshades, grains and dairy. I'm always looking for ways to inspire other parents to cook healthy, nutritious food for the whole family."
CLAIRE HARDING

261

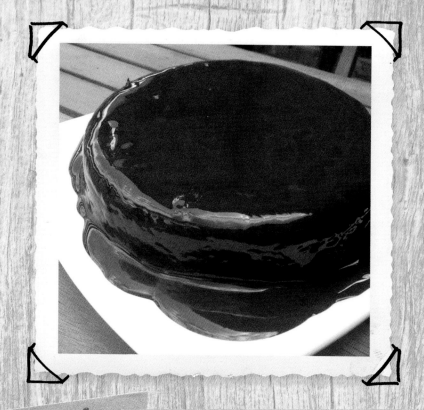

Gran's Chocolate Orange Cake

Ingredients

★ 1 orange
★ 4 eggs
★ 1 cup (220g) ground almonds
★ ¾ cup (170g) raw honey, maple syrup, coconut palm sugar or cane sugar
★ 1 tsp baking soda

FOR THE CHOCOLATE GANACHE

★ 5 ounces (150g) 70-85% cacao
★ 7 tbsp (100ml) double cream

1 Bring a saucepan of water to boil and place the orange in the pan. Bring to a simmer and cook for around 60 minutes until soft. Remove from the water and allow to cool.

2 Preheat the oven to 325°F.
Line a cake pan with parchment paper and a little butter or olive oil, or use baking/muffin cups. (Grease these a little too to prevent them from sticking.)

3 Whisk the eggs and sweetener of your choice in a food processor until thick and pale. Add the ground almonds, cooked orange (the whole orange, peel included) and baking soda to the processor and mix again until the ingredients have blended thoroughly and there are no large lumps of orange.

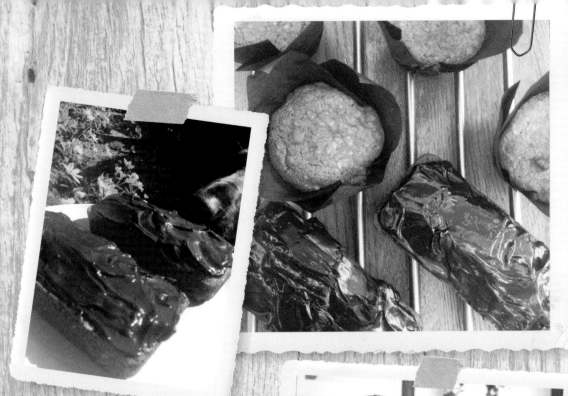

4 Spoon the cake mixture into the prepared cake tray. If making muffins, bake in the oven for 25-30 minutes. If making a cake, bake for 50 minutes. Check by inserting a clean knife. If the knife comes out dry, the cakes are ready. Remove from the oven and allow to cool. Once cooled, remove from the pan/cups.

5 To make the ganache, melt the chocolate in a bowl over a saucepan of boiling water, then add the cream and mix thoroughly. Pour the ganache over the cooled cake and then place in the fridge to allow the ganache to set.

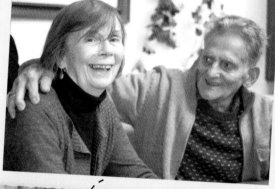

"This is one of the most popular cakes on our Fitter Food website, and we have to credit Keris's grandma Audrey with the recipe. She served up this cake at a family party long before the paleo diet was even thought of." KERIS'S GRANDMA, AUDREY

MAKES:
14 muffins, or the cake serves 10

PREP TIME
1 hour (to boil the orange)
15 minutes

COOKING TIME
Muffins 25-30 minutes
Cake 50 minutes

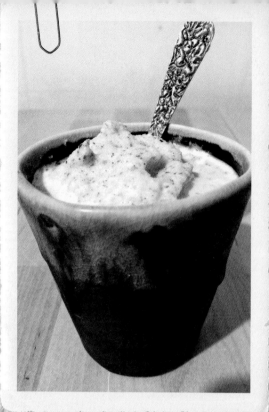

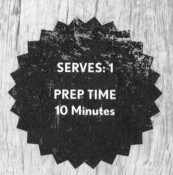

Emma's Almond Granite

Ingredients

★ 4 tbsp (50g) ground almonds
★ 3 tbsp (40g) xylitol
★ 10 drops of almond extract
★ 1 egg white
★ ½ cup (120g) ice cubes

1 Place the almonds, xylitol, almond extract and egg whites in a food processor and blend until it forms a paste.

2 Blend the almond paste with ½ cup (120g) ice cubes or crushed ice to make an iced drink.

I'm a naturopath and owner of Emma Mihill Nutrition. I often collaborate with Fitter Food on nutrition education projects. We've also become great friends and just love hanging out and eating great food together. I've just returned from Sicily where I came across Mandorla Granite, a traditional dish made with almonds. I gave it a healthy twist!" EMMA

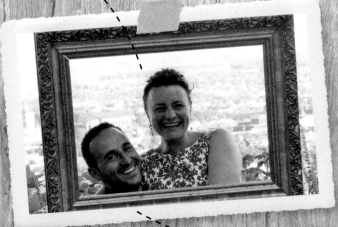

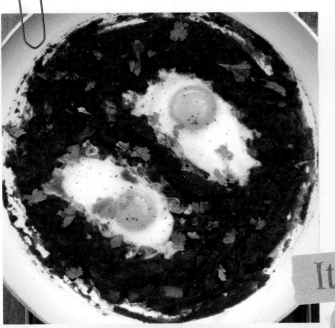

SERVES: 6

PREP TIME
10 Minutes

COOKING TIME
20 Minutes

Dan's Italian Eggs and Sauce

Ingredients

★ 4 eggs
★ 2 tbsp olive oil
★ 1 small to medium onion, finely chopped
★ 2 cloves garlic, peeled and finely chopped
★ 1 can chopped tomatoes
★ 1-1/4 cup (300ml) sauce
★ 3 tbsp tomato purée
★ 3 tbsp xylitol or coconut palm sugar (this takes away the acidity of the tomatoes, so my Nonna used to say)
★ Celtic Sea or Himalayan Pink salt and freshly ground black pepper

"I'm Italian and traditionally this sauce would be made a day in advance for pasta and the leftovers used to bake eggs. However, since my wife Emma is a naturopath and always on about this gluten-free malarkey I mainly just have the eggs 'n' sauce bit. I served it to Keris and Matt for brunch topped with Parma ham. They loved it and asked me to share the recipe." DAN

THE ITALIAN SAUCE

1 Heat the olive oil in a pan on medium heat before adding the onion and garlic, stirring and cooking for about 5 minutes until the onions soften.

2 Add the canned tomatoes, sauce, tomato purée and mix together; then add the xylitol or sugar, salt and pepper. Stir again, then bring to a simmer and cook for 15 minutes or so, stirring occasionally. The longer the sauce cooks, the better, as it develops more flavor that way. If the sauce dries out, add a little water and stir. Taste at this point, and add a little more salt/pepper/sugar if you think it's necessary. Tasting at this point is key—your tongue won't lie!

THE EGGS & SAUCE

1 Add the desired amount of sauce to cover the base of a small-to-medium frying pan and warm the sauce on a low heat.

2 Make small wells in the sauce and crack the desired amount of eggs into the sauce. Don't break the yolk.

3 Poach the egg in the sauce and carefully spoon the hot sauce on top of the egg. This helps to cook the yolk at the same time as the egg white is being cooked beneath. Top with fresh herbs of your choice and enjoy.

265

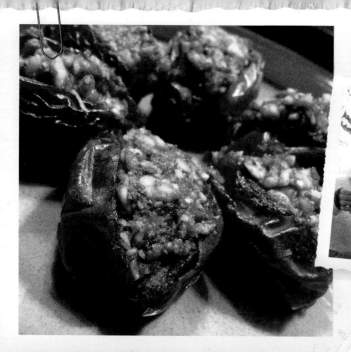

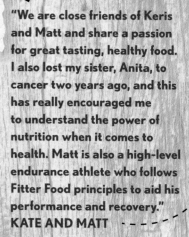

"We are close friends of Keris and Matt and share a passion for great tasting, healthy food. I also lost my sister, Anita, to cancer two years ago, and this has really encouraged me to understand the power of nutrition when it comes to health. Matt is also a high-level endurance athlete who follows Fitter Food principles to aid his performance and recovery."
KATE AND MATT

Kate and Matt's Fancy a (Fancier!) Date?

Ingredients

★ 6 large medjool dates
★ 1/4 cup (50g) pistachios, unshelled, unsalted
★ Grated rind of 1 orange
★ 1 tbsp orange juice
★ 2 tsp raw honey
★ ¼ tsp cinnamon
★ ¼ tsp nutmeg
★ 1 pinch ground cloves
★ 1 pinch Celtic Sea or Himalayan Pink salt

1 Make a slice lengthways in each date and remove the stone (but don't cut all the way through!)

2 Add all remaining ingredients to food processor and process until blended and the nuts are finely chopped.

3 Stuff some pistachio mixture into each date.

4 Enjoy with a cup of tea.

SERVES: 6

**PREP TIME
10 Minutes**

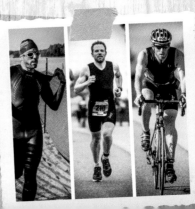

Thai Coconut Shrimp Cakes with Tangy Cilantro Sauce

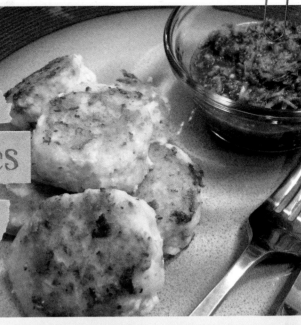

Ingredients

COCONUT SHRIMP CAKES

★ 2 shallots, roughly chopped
★ 1 clove garlic, roughly chopped
★ 1 pound (400g) raw peeled shrimp
★ 1 tbsp coconut flour
★ 1 tbsp desiccated coconut
★ 1 pinch nutmeg
★ 1 egg
★ Celtic Sea or Himalayan Pink salt and freshly ground black pepper
★ 1 small green chili, roughly chopped (optional)
★ Small handful cilantro leaves (optional)
★ Coconut oil (for frying)

CILANTRO SAUCE

★ 1 green chili, de-seeded and roughly chopped
★ 1 green pepper, de-seeded and roughly chopped
★ Half a thumb of ginger, peeled and chopped
★ 2 cloves garlic, roughly chopped
★ Large handful cilantro, stalks removed, roughly chopped
★ 1 tsp coconut palm sugar
★ 2 tsp white rice vinegar
★ Juice of a lemon
★ Celtic Sea or Himalayan Pink salt and freshly ground black pepper

A great dinner party starter, as it can be prepped ahead and takes just a couple of minutes to cook.

1 If shrimp is frozen, defrost in cool water for 15 minutes before using. Blend shrimp cake ingredients in a food processor until well mixed. Shape into 10-12 cakes and chill for a couple of hours or overnight.

2 When ready to use, heat coconut oil in a pan and fry for around 5 minutes on each side until browned and fully cooked.

3 While the shrimp cakes are chilling, make the sauce by blending all the ingredients together in a food processor. Place in a bowl and chill until ready to serve.

MAKES:
4 Fishcakes

PREP TIME
15 Minutes

COOKING TIME
10 Minutes

267

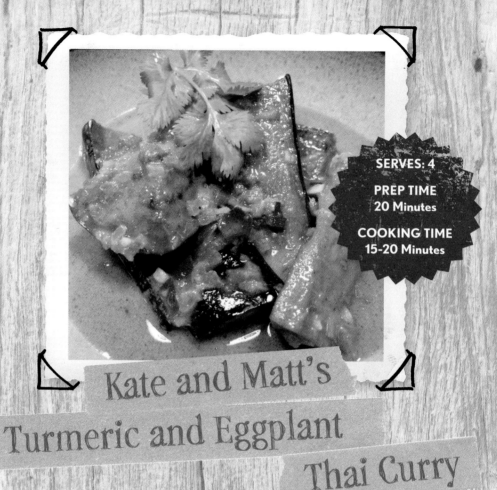

Kate and Matt's Turmeric and Eggplant Thai Curry

Ingredients

2 medium/large eggplant

2 tbsp ground turmeric

1 tsp chili powder

2 red chilis, de-seeded and roughly chopped

5 cloves garlic, roughly chopped

6 shallots, roughly chopped

Thumb of fresh ginger, peeled and chopped

1 tbsp Thai fish sauce

1 tbsp coconut palm sugar

1 tbsp coconut oil

1 can coconut milk

¾ cup (200ml) vegetable stock

Celtic Sea or Himalayan Pink salt and freshly ground black pepper

Fresh cilantro to serve

1 Quarter the eggplant lengthways and chop each in half again (crossways). Mix the turmeric and chili powder in a bowl. Coat the eggplant pieces on all sides with the turmeric and chili mixture.

2 Put the chili, garlic, ginger, shallots, fish sauce and palm sugar in a food processor and blend into a finely chopped, rough paste.

3 Heat the coconut oil in a frying pan, add the eggplant pieces and brown on all sides. Remove to a plate. Now add the chili, garlic, ginger and shallot mixture to the pan and fry for a couple of minutes.

4 Add the eggplant pieces back into the pan, along with the coconut milk and stock. Mix and bring to a boil. Then simmer for around 15 minutes. The dish is ready when the eggplant is soft but still holds its shape.

5 Season to taste and serve with a sprinkling of chopped fresh cilantro.

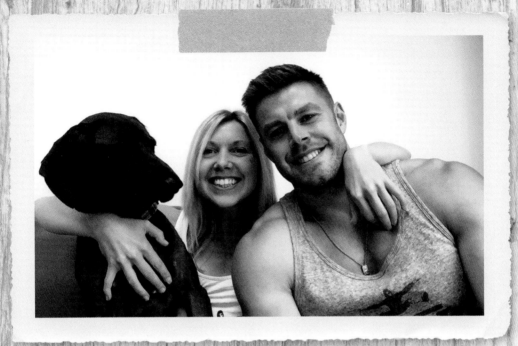

We'd like to thank you for buying our book. It really means the world to us and we're grateful you chose to invest in a taste of Fitter Food.

We genuinely hope this becomes your kitchen bible and you enjoy cooking the recipes for yourself and your friends and family on a regular basis.

BOSH!

Keris, Matt and Hamish

NUTRITIONAL INFORMATION

Eating Fitter Food doesn't require that you count calories. However, we know some people like to track their daily intake of carbohydrates and dietary fats. With that in mind, we offer the following nutritional values. But unlike processed foods that are produced by machines, home cooking macronutrient measurements are not entirely exact. For one, fresh produce tends to come in various sizes. And it may be that you chose a larger fish fillet or steak, a larger serving of greens or you decide to be less liberal with the sweetener. To that end, the following nutritional values are estimates, gathered from various online resources.

All the recipes are calculated for single portions. In recipes that state a range—say "1 to 2 teaspoons of a specific herb," or "serves 4 to 5 people"—we have chosen to calculate the more caloric option. **So these macronutrients may be lower if you chose to serve a greater number of people**.

	CALORIES	CARBS (G)	PROTEIN (G)	FAT (G)
BREAKFAST				
English Breakfast Frittata	475	6	33	37
Avocado and Salmon Calzone	256	3	20	18
Protein Pancakes	312	32	25	9
Sweet Pot Pancakes (per pancake)	99	8	3	6
Chia Banana Porridge	564	57	8	36
Brunch Loaf (based on 4 servings)	270	5	20	18
Omega to Go Muffins (per muffin)	163	2	16	10
Sweet Potato Hash Browns (per hash brown)	211	21	6	12
Raspberry and Apple Power Oatmeal	362	43	26	8
Chocolate Ready Brekkie	535	68	29	19
Eggs in Avo Boats	379	8	29	29
Fitter Breakfast Wraps (per wrap)	238	41	6	5
Big Breakfast ZZZ Bake	488	30	24	33
One Pan Breakfast	481	10	22	31
Piggy Pots	219	2	20	15
Cottage Flaxcakes	388	4	26	29
Salty Banana Cinnamon Scramble	300	30	14	15
Turkey Toast Toppers	303	4	39	14

	CALORIES	CARBS (G)	PROTEIN (G)	FAT (G)
SMOOTHIES				
Mint Choc Chip	141	23	10	3
Choc Avo Bliss	341	49	13	14
Hidden Greens	325	31	24	15
Carrot and Mango	296	36	11	15
Green Machine	179	19	12	7
Banana Bread	421	46	25	17
Kale Chocolate Ginger	146	22	10	3
Coconut Greens	344	25	24	18
SOUPS				
Carrot and Apple	238	19	4	16
Hulk	207	23	10	9
Carrot Cumin and Ginger	238	35	9	8
Chili Chicken and Tomato	118	11	4	6
Sweet Potato and Kale	109	20	5	2
Creamy Broccoli, Kale and Ginger	271	18	8	19
Tomato and Tarragon	238	22	9	14
Minty Zucchini	121	10	5	7
MEALS IN MINUTES				
Fish				
Fish In a Mediterranean Bag	191	9	17	10
Fish In a Caribbean Bag	391	4	64	11
Fish In a Thai Bag	202	8	17	11
Stir Fried Shrimp with Cauliflower Rice	202	14	18	8
Smoked Salmon and Squash Frittata	254	15	18	14
(based on 8 slices)				
Marinated Garlic, Honey and Mustard Salmon	384	11	29	25
Seafood Tandoori Mixed Grill	298	5	35	15
Simple Spanish Omelet	203	7	15	12
Quick Seafood Stir Fry	182	11	22	5
Citrus Salmon with Pea and Avocado Mash	401	23	37	18
Easy Shrimp Red Thai Curry	240	10	8	7
Tomato, Caper and Olive Salmon	367	18	49	11
Fish, Chips and Mushy Pea Cakes	227	31	54	4
Paella Pronto	527	27	41	13

	CALORIES	CARBS (G)	PROTEIN (G)	FAT (G)
Fish (Cont.)				
Fish in Parsley Sauce	433	7	19	45
Curried Fish Bake	229	14	21	10
Poultry				
Chicken Tandoori Skewers	441	15	47	23
Chicken Fajitas	224	16	21	7
Tamari, Ginger and Lime Chicken	407	2	38	27
Pesto Chicken with Zucchini	456	17	27	33
Pimped Up Peri Peri Chicken	241	4	22	15
Thigh Thai Green Curry	415	30	3	35
Spanish Style Chicken (Using Sweet Potatoes)	417	42	43	8
Crispy Chicken in Tarragon Sauce	471	13	46	28
Mini Protein Pizzas	305	3	25	21
Meat				
Zucchini Carbonara	338	2	21	27
Thai Steak Style Salad	473	34	51	16
Beef 5 A Day Stir Fry	325	24	20	16
Mexican Style Scotch Eggs (per Scotch egg)	348	2	29	25
Moroccan Style Meatballs	479	12	31	33
Italian Style Scotch Eggs (per Scotch egg)	313	4	22	24
Pork, Apple and Fennel Scotch Eggs (per Scotch egg)	324	6	21	25
Smoky Pork Meatballs	425	15	37	24

	CALORIES	CARBS (G)	PROTEIN (G)	FAT (G)
BURGER SHACK				
Pork, Apple and Leek (serves 5)	209	4	16	14
Lamb, Pea and Mint	315	8	25	20
Greek Salad	213	5	19	13
The Basic Beefy and Cheesy	442	2	31	35
Oriental Pork	239	1	20	17
Pesto Turkey	397	5	24	32
Curry in a Burger	320	1	23	25
Turkey, Chorizo and Red Pepper (serves 6)	279	3	30	17
Smoky Salmon Burgers (serves 4)	383	8	31	25
Greek Style Lamb	428	3	28	34
SOMETHING FOR THE WEEKEND				
Fitter Fish Pie (serves 4)	381	14	43	7
Chicken Kiev	580	17	51	36
Sweet Potato and Lamb Tagine (serves 6)	483	56	36	13
Pulled Pork (serves 6)	649	19	66	33
Spicy Roast Shoulder of Lamb	490	1	46	34
Smoked Salmon and Spinach Frittata	213	5	15	14
Paprika and Almond Crusted Chicken	674	43	15	62
Bosh Bolognese with Zucchini	558	20	47	32
Mediterranean Fish and Chips	306	24	29	11
Bacon and Banana Bread (no maple drizzle)	303	20	12	18
Balsamic Roast Chicken (serves 8)	522	37	81	23
Spicy Ginger Wings (per wing)	87	5	7	5
Butternut Squash Lasagna (serves 8)	437	25	26	27
Sweet Potato Chocolate Chili	589	32	34	33
Sticky Pork Spare Ribs (per rib)	230	15	17	11
Veggie Fest Curry (serves 8)	252	25	6	15
SIDES				
Pimped Up Pesto Potatoes	330	31	8	21
Sweet Patatas Bravas	436	72	9	8

	CALORIES	CARBS (G)	PROTEIN (G)	FAT (G)
SALADS				
Steak and Halloumi Salad (no pesto)	565	41	3	43
Goji Green Salad	301	13	35	10
Chicken Cumin and Orange Salad	556	41	23	33
Epic Herby Salad	163	20	5	8
Cheesy Zucchini Chips	247	7	11	19
Sticky Coconut Mango Rice	502	68	8	25
Bosh Baked Beans	175	22	8	4
Super Mash	194	41	27	2
Pesto Veghetti	378	12	8	34
Curried Sweet Potato Mash (serves 2)	173	27	4	6
Crinkle-Cut Sesame Sweet Potato Crisps	248	25	3	16
Quick Carrot and Cilantro Slaw	37	7	2	1
SNACKS				
Chicken Squids (per squid)	116	5	6	8
Chocolate Collagen Bites (per bite)	120	7	5	8
Dairy-Free Liver Pate (serves 4)	341	7	39	17
Apricot Energy Shot (per shot)	108	12	4	6
Chocolate Protein Loaf	186	19	15	6
Keen-Wah Energy Bar (per bar)	239	28	6	13
Mini Muscle Cookie (per cookie)	93	4	7	6
Green Tea Muffins (per muffin)	190	17	9	5
Buzz Balls (per ball)	92	4	1	8
Protein Peppermint Thins (per thin)	131	5	6	11
Cream Soda Kefir	16	4	0	0
Speedy Sauerkraut with a Twist	12	5	0.1	1
Crackin' Balls (per ball)	146	3	12	10
Lemon Pepper Mackerel Pate	243	4	16	18
SAUCES, DRESSINGS AND CONDIMENTS				
Cheats Bearnaise Sauce	226	1	1	25
Pimped Guacamole	45	6	1	2
Tartar Sauce	13	1	1	1
Super Simple Ketchup	19	3	0	0
Homemade Pesto	264	4	5	27
Homemade BBQ Sauce	75	12	1	4

	CALORIES	CARBS (G)	PROTEIN (G)	FAT (G)
DESSERTS				
BOSH Brownies (serves 8)	503	34	8	39
Chocolate Ginger Cake (serves 12)	378	23	7	29
Dark Chocolate Delights	223	13	4	18
Carrot, Apple and Sultana Cake	313	20	9	23
Chocolate Beet Cake (serves 8)	345	27	9	24
Microwave Molten Mug Cake	298	29	11	14
Apple Chestnut and Rosemary Loaf	243	29	6	13
S'nickers in a Twist (serves 10)	359	36	5	23
Banana Choc Ices (per choc ice)	171	21	3	9
Post Workout Rice Pudding	375	53	5	17
Funky Monkey Pudding	191	33	4	7
AFTER DINNER BITES				
Aprichoc Balls (serves 24)	126	10	2	9
Bounty Bites (serves 8)	275	14	3	24
BOSH Biscotti (per biscotti half)	187	10	5	15
Goji Protein Truffles	116	5	5	8
FITTER FOOD FAMILY				
Leek, Parsley and Potato Salmon	465	23	59	28
Sweet Potato and Cranberry Cake (serves 8)	435	22	10	29
Paleo Yorkshire Puddings	170	29	4	4
Paleo Bangin' Beef Bulgogi	462	14	30	32
Lil' Balls of Greatness (12 balls)	29	4	1	1
Big Dippers	153	9	6	10
Kefir Garlic and Chive Dip	16	2	1	1
Tarty Nomato Relish	41	8	1	1
Thai Coconut Shrimp Cakes with Tangy Cilantro Sauce (per fishcake)	127	9	17	3
Turmeric and Eggplant Thai Curry	299	30	5	19
Chocolate Orange Cake (serves 10)	354	28	10	25
Almond Granite	419	56	14	25
Italian Eggs and Sauce	217	21	9	12

REFERENCES

1 Blaut, M. & Clavel, T. (2007), "Metabolic Diversity of the Intestinal Microbiota: Implications for Health and Disease," *The Journal of Nutrition* 137 (3): 751S-755S.

2 Kau, A., et al. (2011), "Human nutrition, the gut microbiome, and immune system: envisioning the future," *Nature* 474 (7351): 327-336.

3 USDA National Nutrient Database www.ndb.nal.usda.gov

4 The Human Microbiome Project Consortium (2012) "Structure, function and diversity of the healthy human microbiome." *Nature* 486: 207-214.

5 Spreadbury, I. (2012), "Comparison with ancestral diets suggests dense acellular carbohydrates promote an inflammatory microbiota, and may be the primary dietary cause of leptin resistance and obesity," *Journal of Diabetes, Metabolic Syndrome and Obesity* (5): 175-189.

6 Catherine, A. et al. (2012), "Diversity, stability and resilience of the human gut microbiota," *Nature* 489 (7415): 220-230.

7 Campbell-McBride, N. (2010), *Gut & Psychology Syndrome 2nd Ed*. Norfolk: Medinform.

8 Wald, A. & Adibi, S. (1982), "Stimulation of gastric acid secreted by glycine and related oligopeptides in humans," *American Journal of Physiology* 242 (2): 85-88.

9 Van der Hulst, R., Von Meyenfeldt, M., Soeters, P. (1996) "Glutamine: an essential amino acid for the gut," *Nutrition* 12 (11-12): 78-81.

10 Kresser, C. (2013), "How to Eat More Organ Meats" http://chriskresser.com/how-to-eat-more-organ-meats/ (last accessed 22/10/2015).

11 Conlon, M. & Bird, A. (2015), "The Impact of Diet and Lifestyle on Gut Microbiota and Human Health," *Nutrients* 7 (1): 17-44.

12 Załdski, A., Banaszkiewicz, A., Walkowiak, J. (2013), "Butyric acid in irritable bowel syndrome," *Gastroenterology Review* 8 (6): 350-353.

13 Nakatsuji, T. et al. (2009), "Antimicrobial Property of Lauric Acid Against Propionibacterium Acnes: Its Therapeutic Potential for Inflammatory Acne Vulgaris," *Journal of Investigative Dermatology* 129: 2480-2488.

14 Kresser, C. (2013), "Get rid of heartburn and GERD forever in three simple steps" http://chriskresser.com/get-rid-of-heartburn-and-gerd-forever-in-three-simple-steps/ (last accessed 22/10/2015).

15 Kirpitch, A, & Maryniuk, M. (2011), "The 3 R's of Glycemic Index: Recommendations, Research, and the Real World," Clinical 29 (4): 155-159.

16 Selma, M., Espin, J., Tomas-Barberan, F.A. (2009), "Interaction between phenolics and gut microbiota: Role in human health," *Journal of Agricultural and Food Chemistry* 57: 6485-6500.

17 Wexler, H. (2007), "Bacteroides: the Good, the Bad, and the Nitty-Gritty," *Clinical Microbiology Reviews* 20(4): 593-621.

18 Turnbaugh, P. et al. (2006), "An obesity-associated gut microbiome with increased capacity for energy harvest," *Nature* 444 (7122):1027-31.

19 Marko Kalliomäki, M., Collado, M., Salminen, S., Isolauri, E. (2008), "Early differences in fecal microbiota composition in children may predict overweight," *American Society for Clinical Nutrition* 87 (3): 534-538.

20 Borody, T. & Khoruts, A. (2012), "Fecal microbiota transplantation and emerging applications," *Nature Reviews Gastroenterology and Hepatology* 9: 88-96.

21 US Department of Health & Human Services (2015) Household Products Database. http://householdproducts.nlm.nih.gov/index.htm (last accessed 27 October 2015).

22 www.ewg.org/skindeep/

23 Topping, D., & Clifton, P., (2001), "Short-Chain Fatty Acids and Human Colonic Function: Roles of Resistant Starch and Nonstarch Polysaccharides, *Physiological Reviews* 81(3): 1031-1064.

24 Scott-Dixon, K. & St. Pierre, B. (2015), "Sweet vs. regular potatoes: Which potatoes are really healthier?" http://www.precisionnutrition.com/regular-vs-sweet-potatoes (last accessed 27/10/2015).

25 Landon, S. Coyler, C., Salman, H. (2012), "The Resistant Starch Report: An Australian update on health benefits, measurement and dietary intakes," Food Australia Supplement http://foodaust.com.au/wp-content/uploads/2012/04/Hi_Maize-supplement_web.pdf (last accessed 27/10/2015).

26 Totsch, S., Waite, M., Sorge, R. (2015), "Dietary Influence on Pain via the Immune System," *Progress in Molecular Biology and Translational Science* 131: 435-469.

27 Arreola, R. et al. (2015), "Immunomodulation and anti-inflammatory effects of garlic compounds," *Journal of Immunology Research* vol. 2015 10.1155/2015/401630.

28 Samonina, G. et al. (2000), "Protection of gastric mucosal integrity by gelatin and simple proline containing peptides," *Pathophysiology* 7 (1): 69-73.

29 Blythman, J. (2006) *Bad Food Britain* London: Fourth Estate.

30 Siri-Tarino, P., Sun, Q., Hu, F., Krauss, R., (2010), "Meta-analysis of prospective cohort studies evaluating the association of saturated fat with cardiovascular disease," *American Journal of Clinical Nutrition* 91(3): 535-546.

31 Chowdhury, R. et al. (2014), "Association of Dietary, Circulating, and Supplement Fatty Acids with Coronary Risk: A Systematic Review and Meta-analysis," *Annals of Internal Medicine* 160 (6):398-406.

32 Fernandez, M. (2012), "Rethinking dietary cholesterol," *Current Opinion in Clinical Nutrition and Metabolic Care* 15 (2): 117-121.

33 Djoussé L. & Gaziano J. (2009), "Dietary cholesterol and coronary artery disease: a systematic review," *Current Atherosclerosis Reports* 11(6): 418-422.

34 Available at www.chriskresser.com

35 Alexander, D. & Cushing, C. (2011), "Red meat and colorectal cancer: a critical summary of prospective epidemiologic studies," *Obesity Revolution* 12 (5): 472-493.

36 Belury et al. (2002), "Conjugated linoleic acid is an activator and ligand for peroxisome proliferator-activated receptor-gamma (**PPARγ**)," *Nutrition Research* 22 (7): 817-824.

37 Daley, C. et al. (2010), "A review of fatty acid profiles and antioxidant content in grass-fed and grain-fed beef," *Nutrition Journal* 9:10 http://www.nutritionj.com/content/9/1/10.

38 Jiao, L. et al. (2014), "Dietary consumption of advanced glycation end products and pancreatic cancer in the prospective NIH-AARP Diet and Health Study," *American Journal of Clinical Nutrition* 101 (1): 126-134.

39 Skog., K., Johansson, M., Jägerstad, M., (1998), "Carcinogenic Heterocyclic Amines in Model Systems and Cooked Foods: A Review on Formation, Occurrence and Intake," *Food and Chemical Toxicology* 36 (9-10): 879-896.

40 Jägerstad, M. & Skog K., (2005), "Genotoxicity of heatprocessed foods," *Mutation Research* 574 (1): 156-172.

41 Juraschek, S. et al (2013), "Effect of a High-Protein Diet on Kidney Function in Healthy Adults: Results From the OmniHeart Trial," *American Journal of Kidney Disease* 61 (4): 547-554.

42 Martin, W., Armstrong, L., Rodriguez, N. (2005), "Dietary protein intake and renal function," *Nutrition Metabolism* 2: 25.

43 Juraschek, S. et al (2013), "Effect of a High-Protein Diet on Kidney Function in Healthy Adults: Results From the OmniHeart Trial," *American Journal of Kidney Disease* 61 (4): 547-554.

44 Lindeberg, S, Nilsson-Ehle, P, Terént, A., Vessby, B, Scherstén B. (2004), "Cardiovascular risk factors in a Melanesian population apparently free from stroke and ischaemic heart disease: the Kitava study," *Journal of Internal Medicine* 236 (3): 331-340.

45 Spreadbury, I. (2012), "Comparison with ancestral diets suggests dense acellular carbohydrates promote an inflammatory microbiota, and may be the primary dietary cause of leptin resistance and obesity," *Journal of Diabetes, Metabolic Syndrome and Obesity* (5): 175-189.

46 Morris, C. et al. (2015), "Endogenous circadian system and circadian misalignment impact glucose tolerance via separate mechanisms in humans," *Proceedings of the National Academy of Sciences* 112(17): 2225-2234.

47 Sofer et al. (2013), "Changes in daily leptin, ghrelin and adiponectin profiles following a diet with carbohydrates eaten at dinner in obese subjects," *Nutrition, Metabolism and Cardiovascular Diseases* 23 (8): 744-750.

48 Peuhkuri, K., Sihvola, N., Korpela, R. (2012), "Diet promotes sleep duration and quality," *Nutrition Research* 32 (5): 309-319.

49 Hibbeln, J. et al. (2006), "Healthy intakes of n−3 and n−6 fatty acids: estimations considering worldwide diversity," *American Society for Clinical Nutrition* 83 (6): 1483-1493S.

50 Simopoulos, A., (2008), "The omega-6/omega-3 fatty acid ratio, genetic variation and cardiovascular disease," *Asian Pacific Journal of Clinical Nutrition* 17: 131-134.

51 Kang J., & Liu A., (2013), "The role of the tissue omega-6/omega-3 fatty acid ratio in regulating tumor angiogenesis," *Cancer Metastasis* 32 (1-2): 201-210.

52 Schurgersa, L. et al. (1999), "Nutritional Intake of Vitamins K1 (Phylloquinone) and K2 (Menaquinone) in The Netherlands," *Journal of Nutritional & Environmental Medicine* 9 (2): 115-122.

53 Nutrition Data http://nutritiondata.self.com/facts/dairyand-egg-products/0/2

54 Larsson, C., Bergkvist, L., Wolk A., (2005), "High-fat dairy food and conjugated linoleic acid intakes in relation to colorectal cancer incidence in the Swedish Mammography Cohort," *American Journal of Clinical Nutrition* 82 (4): 894-900.

55 Kresser, C., (2012), "Shaking Up The Salt Myth: Healthy Salt Recommendations" http://chriskresser.com/shaking-up-the-salt-myth-healthy-salt-recommendations/ (last accessed 22/10/2015).

56 Willett, W. (1998), "Is dietary fat a major determinant of body fat?," *American Journal Of Clinical Nutrition* 67: 556-562.

57 Montmayeur, J., (2010), "Fat Detection: Taste, Texture, and Post Ingestive Effects," http://www.ncbi.nlm.nih.gov/pubmed/21452472

58 Spreadbury, I., (2012), "Comparison with ancestral diets suggests dense acellular carbohydrates promote an inflammatory microbiota, and may be the primary dietary cause of leptin resistance and obesity," Journal of Diabetes, Metabolic Syndrome and Obesity (5): 175-189.

59 Holt, S. et al. (1995), "A satiety index of common foods," *European Journal of Clinical Nutrition* 49 (9): 675-690.

60 Mathieson, RA. et al. (1986), "The effect of varying carbohydrate content of a very-low-caloric diet on resting metabolic rate and thyroid hormones," *Metabolism* 35 (5): 394-398.

61 Lake, A., & Townsend, T. (2006), "Obesogenic environments: exploring the built and food environments," *Journal of the Royal Society for the Promotion of Health* 126 (6): 262-267.

62 Berthoud, H., Lenard, N., Shin, A. (2011), "Food reward, hyperphagia, and obesity," *American Journal of Physiology - Regulatory, Integrative and Comparative Physiology* 300 (6): 1266-1277.

63 Guyenet, S. (2012), "The Potato Diet" http://wholehealthsource.blogspot.co.uk/2012/12/the-potato-diet.html (last accessed 22/10/2015).

64 Hall, K. et al. (2014), "Dynamic Interplay Among Homeostatic, Hedonic, and Cognitive Feedback Circuits Regulating Body Weight," *American Journal of Public Health* 104 (7) 1169-1175.

65 Kasarda, D., Ph.D. (2003), "Celiac Disease and Safe Grains" http://wheat.pw.usda.gov/ggpages/topics/Celiac.vs.grains.html

66 Director of the Mucosal Immunology and Biology Research Center at Mass General Hospital.

67 Fasano, A. (2003), "Prevalence of celiac disease in at-risk and not-at-risk groups in the United States: a large multicenter study," *Archives of Internal Medicine* 163(3): 286-292.

68 Catassi, C. et al. (2013), "Non-Celiac Gluten Sensitivity: The New Frontier of Gluten Related Disorders," *Nutrients* 5(10): 3839-03853.

69 Serena, G., Camhi S., Sturgeon C., Yan S., Fasano A. (2015), "The Role of Gluten in Celiac Disease and Type 1 Diabetes," *Nutrients* 7 (9): 7143-7162.

70 Kresser, C. (2013), "What Are the Hidden Costs of Modern Hygiene?" http://chriskresser.com/what-are-the-hidden-costs-of-modern-hygiene/ (last accessed 22/10/2015).

71 Biesiekierski, J. (2011), "Gluten causes gastrointestinal symptoms in subjects without celiac disease: a double-blind randomized placebo-controlled trial," *The American Journal of Gastroenterology* 106(3): 508-514.

72 Knivsberg, A., Reichelt, K., Høien, T., Nødland, M. (2002), "A randomised, controlled study of dietary intervention in autistic syndromes," *Nutritional Neuroscience* 5 (4): 251-261.

73 Hernandez, M., Colina, G., Ortigosa, L. (1998), "Epilepsy, cerebral calcifications and clinical or subclinical coeliac disease. Course and follow up with gluten-free diet," *Seizure: European Journal of Epilepsy* 7 (1): 49-54.

74 Henry, A, Brooks, A., Piperno, D. (2010), "Microfossils in calculus demonstrate consumption of plants and cooked foods in Neanderthal diets," (Shanidar III, Iraq; Spy I and II, Belgium) *Proceedings of the National Academy of Sciences* 108 (2), 486-491.

75 http://nutritiondata.self.com/facts/dairy-and-eggproducts/0/2

76 Valvoa, M. et al. (2005), "Effect of ewe feeding system (grass v. concentrate) on intramuscular fatty acids of lambs raised exclusively on maternal milk," *Animal Science* 81 (3) pp 431-436.

77 Vojdani, A. & Tarash, I. (2013), "Cross-Reaction between Gliadin and Different Food and Tissue Antigens," *Food Nutrition Sciences* 4 (1) DOI:10.4236/fns.2013.41005.

78 Swallow, D. (2003), "Genetics of lactase persistence and lactose intolerance," *Annual Review of Genetics* 37:197-219.

79 Ho et al. (2014), "Comparative effects of A1 versus A2 beta-casein on gastrointestinal measures: a blinded randomised cross-over pilot study," *European Journal of Clinical Nutrition* 68, 994-1000.

80 Ouwehand, A., Salminen, S., Isolauri, E., (2002), "Probiotics: an overview of beneficial effects," *Antonie van Leeuwenhoek* 82: 279-289.

81 Hoffman, J. & Falvo M., (2004), "Protein - Which is Best?" *Journal of Sports Science and Medicine* 3 (3): 118-130.

82 Lothian, J. Grey, V. Lands, L. (2006), "Effect of whey protein to modulate immune response in children with atopic asthma," *International Journal of Food Sciences and Nutrition* 57 (3-4): 204-211.

83 Bounous, G. (2000), "Whey protein concentrate (WPC) and glutathione modulation in cancer treatment," *Anticancer Research* 20 (6C):4785-4792.

84 Ha, E., Zemel M. (2003), "Functional properties of whey, whey components, and essential amino acids: mechanisms underlying health benefits for active people," *Journal of Nutritional Biochemistry* 14: 251-258.

85 Hoffman, J. & Falvo M., (2004), "Protein - Which is Best?" *Journal of Sports Science and Medicine* 3 (3): 118-130.

86 MacLean, D., Graham, T., Saltin, B. (1994), "Branched-chain amino acids augment ammonia metabolism while attenuating protein breakdown during exercise," *American Journal of Physiology* 267: E1010-1022.

87 Baer, D. et al. (2011), "Whey protein but not soy protein supplementation alters body weight and composition in free-living overweight and obese adults," *Journal of Nutrition* 141(8) 1489-1494.

88 Geiser, M. (2003), "The wonders of whey protein," *NSCA's Performance Training Journal* 2: 13-15.

89 Frankenfield, D., Roth-Yousey, L., Compher, C. (2005), "Comparison of Predictive Equations for Resting Metabolic Rate in Healthy Nonobese and Obese Adults: A Systematic Review," *Journal of the Academy of Nutrition and Dietetics* 105(5): 775-789.

90 Lindeberg et al. (1994), "Cardiovascular risk factors in a Melanesian population apparently free from stroke and ischaemic heart disease: the Kitava study," *Journal of Internal Medicine* 236 (3): 331-340.

91 Biss, K., Taylor, C., Lewis, L., Mikkelson, B., Hussey, L., Jey-Ho K. (1970), "The Masai's protection against atherosclerosis," *Pathology Microbiology* 35(1):198-204.

92 Sofer et al. (2013), "Changes in daily leptin, ghrelin and adiponectin profiles following a diet with carbohydrates eaten at dinner in obese subjects," *Nutrition, Metabolism and Cardiovascular Disease*. 23(8): 744-750.

INDEX

WHO IS BEHIND FITTER FOOD?

Fitter Food was founded by Keris and Matt, two individuals passionate about good food, optimal health, training, and leading long and happy lives. Having a combined experience of over 15 years in the health and fitness industry, they set out on a mission to empower other people with the knowledge and understanding to make the journey to ultimate health.

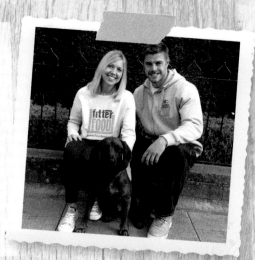

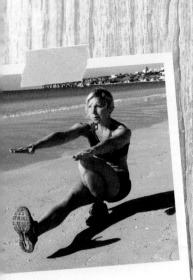

ABOUT KERIS

My health journey still continues to evolve. I started out in the health and fitness industry as a personal trainer, and after experiencing the benefits of daily movement and exercise, I became a little guilty of thinking exercise was the answer to everything. A spell of injuries then led me to revisit the essential role that nutrition and other lifestyle habits play on the road to achieving and maintaining optimal health. As well as eating nutritious food, I now place a much greater focus on sleep and daily stress management. I also walk more than I run these days!

The final piece in my health puzzle was putting this all together into one big **FITTER** lifestyle. This includes lots of time outdoors, prioritizing fun experiences with friends and family, building more robust mental health with mindfulness, and ensuring that my life continues to support my happiness. I believe that this is the key to sustainable health.

In our first book I also discussed my own health battles with Polycystic Ovarian Syndrome, acne, and Irritable Bowel Syndrome and how these experiences led me to explore the medicinal impact of nutrition. I now work full-time as a qualified Naturopathic Nutritional Therapist, using a Functional Medicine approach to help people rebalance their bodies and address a range of health issues including mood disorders, hormone issues, and digestive problems.

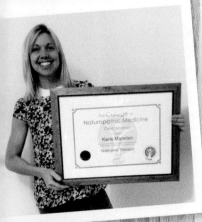

Since the launch of our first book, we've also taken our business online to enable us to reach out and share the Fitter Food message with more and more people. We've coached thousands of people via our nutrition education programs and Fitter 365 Membership site. We use Fitter Food principles, lifestyle power habits, and the support, encouragement and banter of an awesome like-minded community to help people get back to a state of wellness and vitality.

ABOUT MATT

I'm now 30 years old (hard to believe, I know!). I started my training journey at the age of ten, so it has evolved considerably over the years, primarily through making mistakes. These have included over-training, pushing through injuries, and under-valuing the importance of rest and recovery. Because my physique always remained relatively lean, I was also previously under the impression I could eat pretty much whatever I wanted.

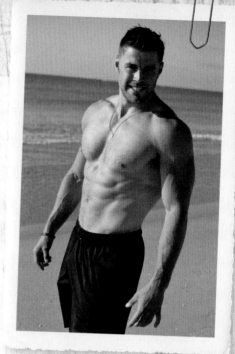

Now I'm a little older (did I mention I'm 30?), and a little wiser. I focus on striking an awesome balance between improving performance in the gym and knowing when to take my foot off the pedal to refocus on stress reduction, improving sleep quality, and of course ensuring that my nutrition supports me on a daily basis. It's a great feeling when you find that balance and have the knowledge required to help you make the right decisions every day. This helps ensure that you thrive as a human being while being able to enjoy the small things in life, which may well include an ice cream and an occasional beer. ☺

I suppose I could use that old saying:

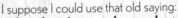

"if only I knew then what I know now."

However, I'm glad I have learned from my mistakes, as it puts me in a great place to help others who are experiencing similar setbacks. I often ask people to reflect on their performance progress, or regression, and consider the bigger picture. This involves listening to their bodies, learning to chill out more, and nourishing themselves with good quality Fitter Food.

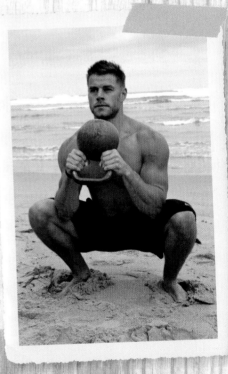

I strive to keep learning every day. One of the biggest milestones for me has been developing a sense of gratitude towards my body; there have certainly been times I've taken it for granted, but now I fully appreciate my ability to perform in the gym and still make strength and skill progressions. Even at my age. ☺ This book is a continuation of our first book. We advocate the same principles and emphasize the same important message:

The Fitter Food message:

You deserve to feel awesome

&

Eating great-tasting and nutritious food is much easier than you think!

Please ensure you read this book from start to finish. Then jump into the kitchen to discover your new favorite recipes. They are all designed to help you hit your goals, and—more importantly—to make you feel happy and healthy.

Health is a voyage of exploration, and we're here to help make it an amazing one!

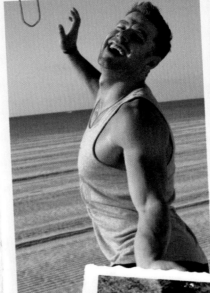

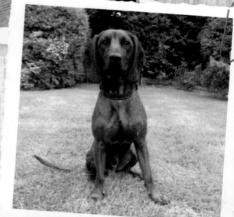

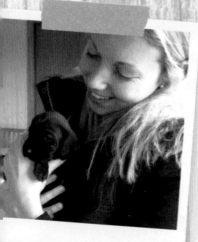

ABOUT HAMISH

Since our last book, there has been a new addition to the Fitter Food family; a Bavarian Mountain Hound called Hamish. Hamish has taught us a huge amount about nutrition, exercise, and healthy lifestyle habits.

By watching him every day, we have come to learn and understand so much about how nature intended us to live. Every morning he wakes up and takes time to do a series of stretches before heading out for a run, walk, or better yet, a sprint. There's simply no agenda to his day, and he does what he feels like. He loves munching on organ meats and bones to make sure he has the nutrients his body needs. He also prioritizes sleep, play and happiness, and loves meeting new people and fellow dogs. In fact, his tail spins if he really likes you!

The icing on the gluten-free Fitter Food cake for many of us should be to **#bemorehamish**. Focus on relaxing a little more, being kinder to our bodies, and listening for feedback when we're tired and stressed out. Often these signals indicate that it's time to ditch the laptop, breathe in some fresh air and head out with our pals for some tail-spinning fun time!

#bemorehamish

JOIN OUR HEALTHY HANGOUT

Fitter 365 is our membership site. It offers a little taste of Fitter Food every single day. It's packed with educational webinars, quick reference guides, exercise videos, gym-based and bodyweight training programs, cooking demonstrations, and all the tools you need to ensure you have the best understanding of health, training and nutrition. The bonus with 365 is the daily interaction and support from the Fitter Food team and a community of like-minded people, all set to answer your questions, have some banter and keep you accountable to your goals, guaranteeing that you get the best possible results.

 Sharon Tait I love the inclusivity and support no matter where you are at in your journey or how big or small your goals are and the ease of the fabulous recipe videos.

Unlike · Reply · 👍3

 Sarah Elizabeth I LOVE the simple, quick and easy recipe ideas for some extra inspiration and the friendly, down-to-earth approach to training and educating the world in the ways of Fitter Food.

Unlike · Reply · 👍7

 Leigh Alliss I've taken part in other online plans and have never felt part of a community the way I do with Fitter Food. The members are supportive and kind and the Fitter Food Team are full of motivation to help you live a healthy life.

Unlike · Reply · 👍4

 Jane Fry Fitter 365 - motivational and life changing - if you want to improve your health, lifestyle and fitness then look no further. Fantastic, sensible advice and fabulous no faff recipes you'll want to cook and share with everyone.

Unlike · Reply · 👍5

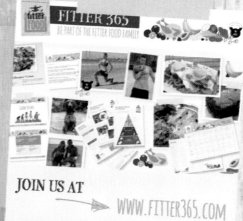

JOIN US AT ➤ WWW.FITTER365.COM

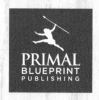

OTHER BOOKS BY PRIMAL BLUEPRINT PUBLISHING

MARK SISSON

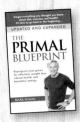

The Primal Blueprint

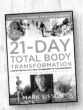

The Primal Blueprint 21-Day Total Body Transformation

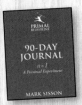

The Primal Blueprint 90-Day Journal: *A Personal Experiment (n=1)*

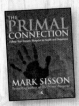

The Primal Connection

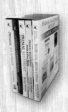

Primal Blueprint Box Set: *Includes the original "Primal Blueprint" hardcover, "The Primal Connection," "The Primal Blueprint Cookbook," "The Primal Blueprint Quick & Easy Meals," and "Primal Blueprint Healthy Sauces, Dressings & Toppings"*

MARK SISSON AND BRAD KEARNS

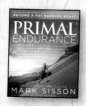 *Primal Endurance*

COOKBOOKS BY MARK SISSON AND JENNIFER MEIER

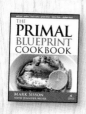 *The Primal Blueprint Cookbook*

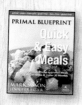 *The Primal Blueprint Quick and Easy Meals*

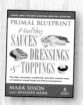 *The Primal Blueprint Healthy Sauces, Dressings, and Toppings*

OTHER AUTHORS

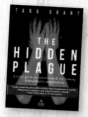

The Hidden Plague
by Tara Grant

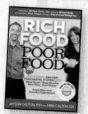

Rich Food, Poor Food
by Mira Calton, CN, and
Jayson Calton, Ph.D.

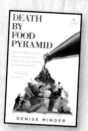

Death by Food Pyramid
by Denise Minger

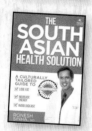

The South Asian Health Solution
by Ronesh Sinha, MD

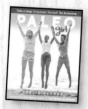

Paleo Girl
by Leslie Klenke

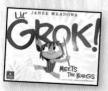

Lil' Grok Meets the Korgs
by Janée Meadows